Responding to Problem Behavior in Schools

The Guilford Practical Intervention in the Schools Series

Kenneth W. Merrell, Series Editor

This series presents the most reader-friendly resources available in key areas of evidence-based practice in school settings. Practitioners will find trustworthy guides on effective behavioral, mental health, and academic interventions, and assessment and measurement approaches. Covering all aspects of planning, implementing, and evaluating high-quality services for students, books in the series are carefully crafted for everyday utility. Features include ready-to-use reproducibles, lay-flat binding to facilitate photocopying, appealing visual elements, and an oversized format.

Recent Volumes

Responding to Problem Behavior in Schools

The Behavior Education Program

SECOND EDITION

DEANNE A. CRONE
LEANNE S. HAWKEN
ROBERT H. HORNER

THE GUILFORD PRESS
New York   London

© 2010 The Guilford Press
A Division of Guilford Publications, Inc.
72 Spring Street, New York, NY 10012
www.guilford.com

Printed in Canada

This book is printed on acid-free paper.

Last digit is print number: 9   8   7   6   5   4   3   2   1

Library of Congress Cataloging-in-Publication Data

Crone, Deanne A.
   Responding to problem behavior in schools : the behavior education program / Deanne A. Crone,
Leanne S. Hawken, Robert H. Horner. — 2nd ed.
      p. cm. — (The Guilford practical intervention in the schools series)
   Includes bibliographical references and index.
   ISBN 978-1-60623-600-0 (pbk.: alk. paper)
   1. Behavior modification—United States.   2. School psychology—United States.   3. Problem
children—Education—United States.   I. Hawken, Leanne S.   II. Horner, Robert
H.   III. Title.
   LB1060.2.C76 2010
   370.15′3—dc22

                                                                                    2009051564

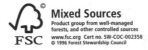

About the Authors

Deanne A. Crone, PhD, is Research Associate at the Center on Teaching and Learning at the University of Oregon. She has directed several research and training grants addressing behavior disorders, positive behavior support, and functional behavioral assessment. Dr. Crone has conducted extensive training in functional behavioral assessment and positive behavior support with teachers, paraprofessionals, principals, and directors of special education.

Leanne S. Hawken, PhD, is Associate Professor in the Department of Special Education at the University of Utah. She has assisted schools in implementing the Behavior Education Program at both the elementary and middle school levels, and has conducted research studies to evaluate its effectiveness. Dr. Hawken's main research focus is positive behavior support, including schoolwide behavior support, targeted interventions for at-risk students, and functional assessment/behavior support planning for students engaging in severe problem behavior.

Robert H. Horner, PhD, is Professor of Special Education at the University of Oregon. He codirects several major research and technical assistance projects addressing positive behavior support. Dr. Horner also has coauthored research assessing the Behavior Education Program approach to behavior support.

Preface

When we published the first edition of this book in 2004, the field of positive behavior support was relatively new, and examples of the extent to which schools were implementing targeted inventions such as the Behavior Education Program (BEP) were scarce. Since the reauthorization of the Individuals with Disabilities Education Act in 2007, schools have been focusing on implementing prevention programs/interventions prior to students needing additional academic or behavior support. To best support all students, a multi-tiered service delivery model termed "response to intervention," or RTI, has been advocated. The goal of the three-tiered RTI model is early identification of students who are at risk for academic challenges due to learning disabilities and provision of an appropriate level of intervention. Researchers in the field of positive behavior support recommend a similar three-tiered model of behavior support to prevent and intervene with serious problem behavior.

Schools across the country are beginning to implement the three-tiered RTI model with documentation of success. There are many examples provided in the literature of how RTI applies to academic behavior (particularly reading), but few models are provided for social behavior. This new edition puts the BEP, a social behavioral intervention, in the context of the three-tiered RTI model and provides detailed step-by-step information on how to implement the intervention. The BEP is one of the few evidence-based Tier II behavior interventions that can support up to 30 students without intensive school personnel time or resources. Many Tier II interventions occur in small groups (e.g., social skills training), resulting in only a small portion of the at-risk population being served. The structure of implementing the BEP schoolwide allows for more students to be served and for schools to free up additional resources to be used with students who need even more intensive behavior support.

In an RTI model, assessment is used for three different purposes: screening, progress monitoring, and diagnostic. This new edition provides details on how to incorporate all three types of assessment while implementing the BEP. First, Chapter 3 describes ways to screen for students who are appropriate for the BEP intervention. Information is provided on how to gather baseline data to further confirm that students who have been screened would likely benefit from the BEP intervention. Key to any RTI model is progress monitoring to quickly determine if the student is benefiting from the intervention. In Chapter 7 we have added detail on how to use student daily progress reports (DPRs) as progress monitoring tools. Diagnostic assessment allows schools to determine how and what to teach. For students who are not responding to the BEP, details are provided in Chapter 8 on how to implement functional behavioral assessment technology to gather diagnostic information. This diagnostic information is then used to modify the BEP to support more students. For students who are not supported by a modified BEP, information is included on what to do if students need more individualized behavior support.

OVERVIEW OF CONTENTS

Overall, the book has been expanded from 7 to 12 chapters. The new edition includes special considerations for high school as well as preschool populations. Critical to the success of the BEP is effective adaptation to the culture of each school and to the culture of the student populations served. New to this edition is a chapter on cultural considerations (Chapter 11), which examines the extent to which school personnel are implementing culturally responsive behavior interventions, including the BEP.

Chapter 1 provides an overview of the critical components of the BEP and a discussion of which schools may be interested in implementing this program. In addition, this chapter briefly introduces the companion DVD, "The Behavior Education Program: A Check-In, Check-Out Intervention for Students at Risk."

Chapter 2 details how the BEP fits into a school's overall behavior support system as a Tier II targeted intervention. New to this edition are the key features of Tier II interventions along with examples of different Tier II interventions. Schools should have several Tier II interventions available, and this chapter discusses the advantages for including the BEP as one type of Tier II intervention. When the previous edition was published, few studies had been conducted documenting the effectiveness of the BEP. This chapter provides an updated summary of the research on the BEP and similar check-in, check-out interventions.

Chapter 3 provides the nuts and bolts of how to implement the BEP intervention, and in this edition includes an extensive discussion of which students are appropriate for the BEP and how to identify students for the intervention. From our work across the country, the biggest errors we saw schools making involved implementing the BEP with students who were already engaging in severe problem behavior. We know from the research summarized in Chapter 2 that the students who benefit most are those *at risk* for developing serious problem behavior, and this chapter outlines how to best identify those students. Key to determining students' responses to intervention is getting baseline data and comparing those data to how students respond postintervention. This chapter includes a discussion of how to gather baseline data to allow for pre–post comparisons of DPR data.

Chapter 4 provides a detailed description of how to successfully introduce and implement the BEP schoolwide. There is a description of how to encourage faculty commitment, including when and how the BEP DVD (mentioned above) should be shown to staff, and the chapter also includes "The BEP Development and Implementation Guide." To design the BEP to fit the needs and culture of your schools, behavior support teams should set aside at least one professional development day and answer all the questions in this guide prior to piloting the BEP.

Much of the content in Chapter 5 has been updated and expanded. This chapter provides a more in-depth look at not only the roles and responsibilities of each person in the school who will be involved in BEP implementation (e.g., BEP coordinator, teacher, behavior support team), but also provides a summary of the training needs for everyone involved, including parents. Many figures have been added to this chapter that detail "scripts" of phrases the BEP coordinator can say at check-in and check-out, as well as sample statements teachers can make when providing feedback to students.

All of the material in Chapter 6 is new and provides school teams with guidelines on how to effectively develop a DPR to fit their school culture. Included is information regarding ranking systems, number of rating periods, and other essential information that should be considered when designing a DPR. New information is provided on how to develop an effective reinforcement system to implement with the BEP. Sample reinforcement systems are also provided, along with a tool for assessing reinforcer preference with older students.

Chapter 7 presents new information on how to measure response to BEP implementation. Specifically, schools are given examples of data that can be easily tracked pre- and post-BEP implementation. New since the first edition is the web-based information system titled "Check-In, Check-Out," or CICO, which is embedded in the School-Wide Information System (SWIS). This system allows for schools to track both office discipline referrals and BEP DPR data. Chapter 7 also details how to collect fidelity of implementation data along with strategies to fade students from the BEP intervention.

Chapter 8 provides strategies for adapting the BEP when students are not responding to the intervention. This information has been updated and expanded from the previous edition. School teams are given tools to use functional behavioral assessment to adapt and/or modify the BEP to support more students. A section is also included about how to include a student with an individualized education plan in the BEP intervention and factors that should be considered.

New to this edition, Chapter 9 gives readers a summary of the adaptations that are necessary to implement the BEP in high school settings. The chapter includes information on selecting students for the intervention, the daily features of the BEP, and how to combine the social aspect of the BEP intervention with the needed academic supports at the high school level. Information is also provided on how to evaluate intervention effectiveness. Implementing the BEP in high school settings is relatively new, and this chapter includes a recent case study evaluation.

Chapter 10, also new to this edition, provides information on how to adapt the BEP to preschool settings. The chapter begins with a rationale for why preschools should consider implementing the BEP. Next, information is provided on how the key features of the BEP can be adapted to be more developmentally appropriate for younger students. Included are a table comparing the BEP for elementary and middle school settings with the preschool BEP and a sample DPR. Finally, the chapter includes a case example to provide details on how the daily, weekly, and monthly features of the BEP could be implemented in preschool settings.

As previously noted, Chapter 11 covers cultural considerations related to implementing the BEP. The chapter begins with a brief definition of culturally competent interventions, then details how school staff should examine their own behavior in relation to interacting with students from different ethnic, cultural, socioeconomic, and religious backgrounds. Case examples are included throughout the chapter to detail how the BEP can be modified to support students from diverse backgrounds. Information is provided about how to evaluate the extent to which the BEP and other behavior interventions are working in schools to ensure they support all students.

Chapter 12 answers frequently asked questions related to implementing the BEP. This chapter has been updated and expanded based on our work across the country and the many questions that have come up in our workshops and inservice trainings. In helping schools implement the BEP, we have learned the signs that indicate that the BEP will not be implemented correctly or that implementation will suffer, such as use of the BEP as a punishment system rather than as a positive behavior support system. We have presented these as precorrections to ensure that school personnel can be successful in implementing the BEP.

This new edition attempts to respond to questions and challenges experienced by schools across the country that used the first edition to build a Tier II level system of positive behavior support for their students. We hope the new and revised material in this edition increases the relevance, feasibility, and functionality of the BEP for schools that begin or continue implementation of the program in coming years.

ACKNOWLEDGMENTS

We extend appreciation and credit to the faculty, staff, and students of Fern Ridge Middle School, Meadowview Elementary, Bohemia Elementary, Vista Elementary, Mountain View Elementary, Academy Park Elementary, Bethel School District, and Tigard–Tualatin School District for their innovations, suggestions, implementation efforts, and encouragement in the development of this book. A special thank you to Mishele Carroll in Granite School District, who developed several forms and some content presented in this book. We would like to acknowledge Dr. Don Kincaid and Dr. Doug Cheney for providing feedback and suggestions on revisions to include in this edition. We thank our contributing authors, Sandra MacLeod, Jessica Swain-Bradway, Susan Johnston, Joan Schumann, and Jason Burrow-Sánchez, for their valuable contributions to this second edition. We would also like to thank Rob March for his contributions to the initial research on the BEP. Finally, thank you to all the school staff across the country who have shared their enthusiasm for the BEP and provided many suggestions during our workshops and training sessions.

Contents

4. Getting a BEP Intervention Started   39

5. Roles, Responsibilities, and Training Needs Related   49
to Implementing the BEP

DEANNE A. CRONE, LEANNE S. HAWKEN, and K. SANDRA MACLEOD

CHAPTER 1

Introduction to the Behavior Education Program

WHAT IS THE PURPOSE OF THE BOOK?

The purpose of this book is to describe a targeted system of positive behavior support called the Behavior Education Program (BEP): what it is, how it works, who can benefit from it, how it is implemented in a school, and how it can be adapted to meet the needs of certain groups or individuals. The goal of the book is to provide the reader with the rationale, procedures, and tools to (1) determine if a BEP system is appropriate for your school, and (2) implement a variation of the BEP that fits the needs of your school.

The BEP is intended to be one piece of the larger behavior support effort in a school. Schools that have effective and complete systems of positive behavior support in place address three levels of behavioral need:

1. Universal support (Tier I): All students must be taught the schoolwide rules and expectations, and teachers must have proactive classroom management procedures in place.
2. Targeted group interventions (Tier II): Students who are at risk of developing patterns of problem behavior must have a system for reducing problem behavior before it becomes worse over time.
3. Individualized student interventions (Tier III): Students with serious problem behavior must receive intensive, individualized behavior support.

The BEP addresses the second level of behavioral need. (For resources on the first and third levels of behavioral need, refer to the Resources section at the end of Chapter 2.) The BEP is designed for students who demonstrate persistent problem behavior in classroom settings, but not dangerous or violent behavior. These are students who do not respond well to schoolwide behavioral expectations, nor to preventative classroom management practices. These are *not* students with serious, chronic behavior problems who require comprehensive, individualized interventions. *A primary function of the BEP is to improve the overall efficiency of the schoolwide procedures, while reducing the number of individualized interventions that are needed.*

Resources in schools are dwindling or being drastically cut. At the same time, schools are expected to do more to support students with diverse academic, emotional, and behavioral needs. This book provides teachers, administrators, school psychologists, educational assistants, and other school personnel with the tools to implement an *efficient* and *cost-effective* system of positive behavior support in their schools. The book details the logic, procedures, administrative systems, and forms needed to build a BEP system. Tools for ongoing evaluation and improvement of the system are also provided. A list of acronyms and definitions appears in Appendix A.1 for a quick review of terms, as needed.

WHAT IS THE BEP?

The BEP is a school-based program for providing daily support and monitoring to students who are at risk for developing serious or chronic problem behavior. Students who fail to respond to schoolwide approaches and who receive several office disciplinary referrals (ODRs) per year may benefit from a Tier II intervention like the BEP. It is based on a daily check-in/check-out system that provides the student with immediate feedback on his or her behavior (via teacher rating on a Daily Progress Report [DPR]) and increased positive adult attention. Behavioral expectations are clearly defined, and students are given both immediate and delayed reinforcement for meeting those expectations. Collaboration between the school and the families of identified students is encouraged by daily sending home a copy of the DPR to be signed by the parents or caregivers and brought back the next school day. A critical feature of the BEP is the use of data to evaluate its effectiveness in changing student behavior. Points earned on the DPR are recorded on a summary graph for each student. These data are reviewed by the school's behavior support team, at least every 2 weeks, and are used to make decisions whether to continue, modify, or fade the BEP intervention.

The BEP incorporates several core principles of positive behavior support, including (1) clearly defined expectations, (2) instruction on appropriate social skills, (3) increased positive reinforcement for following expectations, (4) contingent consequences for problem behavior, (5) increased positive contact with an adult in the school, (6) improved opportunities for self-management, and (7) increased home–school collaboration.

The BEP goes beyond its impact on a single student. It provides the school with a proactive, preventive approach to recurrent problem behavior. In addition, the BEP intervention enhances communication among teachers, improves school climate, increases consistency among staff, and helps teachers to feel supported.

HOW EFFICIENT AND COST-EFFECTIVE IS THE BEP?

The BEP is continuously available, can be implemented within 3–5 days of identifying a problem, and typically requires no more than 5–10 minutes per teacher per day. Although additional coordination time is required, this system can be used by all teachers and staff in a school, with low time demands. All staff are trained to implement the BEP intervention, which is available for students who need additional positive behavior support. Unlike intensive, individualized interventions (i.e., those requiring a functional behavioral assessment [FBA] and an intensive behavior support plan), no lengthy assessment process is conducted prior to the student receiving BEP support. A student who is referred for the BEP intervention can be deemed an appropriate candidate and begin to receive support within 3–5 school days. Personnel time required to implement the intervention is minimal (see Chapter 5 for resource and time requirements), and many students (20–30) can be supported on the system at the same time. Implementation and maintenance costs are low (see Chapter 4 for an example budget).

WHY ARE TIER II
INTERVENTIONS LIKE THE BEP NECESSARY?

Most schools do not have the time or resources to provide comprehensive individualized behavior support for *all* students who need varying levels of extra support. For example, in a school with a population of 500 students, it is estimated that approximately 15–20%, or 75–100 students, will need more support than what schoolwide prevention efforts provide. Conducting intensive, individualized interventions with all of these students would be unmanageable and would tax school resources beyond capacity. Many students will successfully respond to simple intervention strategies, like the BEP, that are less time-intensive and more cost-efficient to implement. Thus, utilizing a program like the BEP will reduce the overall number of students who need individualized support.

Implementing the BEP system in your school does not negate the need to provide intensive, individualized interventions to some students. There will be students for whom the BEP will not be adequate to produce significant reductions in problem behavior. For those students, an FBA should be conducted, and data from the assessment should be used to develop an individualized behavior support plan. (For more information on intensive, individualized positive behavior support, refer to Crone & Horner, 2003.)

WHICH SCHOOLS SHOULD CONSIDER IMPLEMENTING THE BEP?

Schools that have a schoolwide system of positive behavior support (Lewis & Sugai, 1999; Sugai & Horner, 2002a) in place and that still have 10 or more students needing extra support should consider implementing the BEP. A schoolwide system of positive behavior support clarifies expectations both for students and staff, thus reducing the overall number of students engaging in problem behavior. If there are fewer than 10 students who engage in problem behavior, a school may be able to simply implement individualized behavior supports for each of them, rather than invest in the BEP.

Although the BEP is cost-effective and requires minimal staff time, the sincere commitment of *all* staff members and the support of the building administrator are crucial to the success of the program. Administrator support includes the allocation of personnel time and resources to implementation, coordination, and ongoing evaluation of the intervention. Chapter 4 details the steps necessary to get the BEP started in your school and includes a self-assessment checklist to determine readiness for implementing the intervention system.

"IF MY SCHOOL IS ALREADY IMPLEMENTING A SYSTEM LIKE THE BEP FOR AT-RISK STUDENTS, WILL I STILL BENEFIT FROM READING THIS BOOK?"

Yes! This book may help you improve the efficiency of your BEP-type intervention, or help you impose an organizing structure that you may currently lack. Additionally, in Chapter 8, we discuss adaptations and elaborations of the BEP intervention that may help you identify effective modifications to be used when the basic BEP is inadequate for a particular student.

Furthermore, many schools have a program(s) in place to support students who have difficulty meeting academic and behavioral expectations. Often, however, students are placed into these programs without attention to the reason behind the student's problem behavior. *Is the curriculum material too difficult for the student? Does the student act out to get a reaction from his peers? Does the student like staying in from recess and getting one-to-one adult attention when he or she hasn't finished his or her classwork?*

This book describes a brief assessment process to help school personnel think "functionally" about problem behavior, that is, to determine the reason for a student's problem behavior. If a student repeatedly engages in a problem behavior, a pattern will likely emerge. These patterns of behavior can be manipulated to decrease inappropriate behavior while increasing desired behavior. This brief assessment and intervention process is discussed in Chapter 8.

"ARE THERE ADDITIONAL RESOURCES TO AID IMPLEMENTATION OF THE BEP IN MY SCHOOL?"

Yes! A primary resource that schools use in tandem with this book is a DVD titled *The Behavior Education Program: A Check-In Check-Out Intervention for Students at Risk* (Hawken, Pettersson, Mootz, & Anderson, 2005), which is available for purchase at *www.guilford.com*. This DVD outlines the essential features of the BEP and provides video examples of effective BEP implementation. Chapter 5 describes how and when the BEP DVD could be used as a training resource for your school staff. Finally, additional resources are recommended at the end of various chapters throughout this book.

CHAPTER 2

The Context for
Positive Behavior Support in Schools

Schools face a growing challenge in meeting both the instructional and behavioral needs of all students. Students today present with diverse needs and present educators with a unique set of challenges (e.g., English as second language, difficulties associated with low socioeconomic status [SES], significant learning and behavioral needs; Tyack, 2001). To be effective in supporting all students, schools need to implement a continuum of positive behavior support, from less intensive to more intensive, based on the severity of the problem behavior presented (Walker et al., 1996). This continuum includes positive behavior support at three levels: (1) Tier I, schoolwide positive behavior support strategies; (2) Tier II interventions for students at risk; and (3) Tier III interventions for students engaging in severe problem behavior. The continuum of positive behavior support is detailed in Figure 2.1.

The triangle represents all students in the school and is divided into three levels of intervention. The bottom part of the triangle represents the approximately 80% of students who will benefit from primary-level interventions (Colvin, Kameenui, & Sugai, 1993; Sugai & Horner, 1999; Taylor-Greene et al., 1997). Tier I interventions are implemented with all students, in all settings, and include two components: (1) implementing a schoolwide positive behavior support (PBS) plan and (2) implementing proactive classroom behavior management strategies. A school that implements schoolwide PBS (1) generates staff agreement on three to five positively stated rules or expectations, (2) instructs students on the expectations, (3) provides reinforcement for following expectations, (4) provides minor consequences for rule infractions, and (5) uses data on a regular basis to determine whether the schoolwide behavior plan is working. We recommend that schools must have an effective and well-established schoolwide PBS plan in place *prior* to implementing the BEP. In addition, it is important for teachers to utilize effective classroom management practices prior to implementing the BEP.

Once Tier I interventions are in place, we recommend the addition of a Tier II intervention system to support students who continue to engage in frequent problem behavior. In the triangle, the middle portion represents the approximately 15% of students who will benefit from

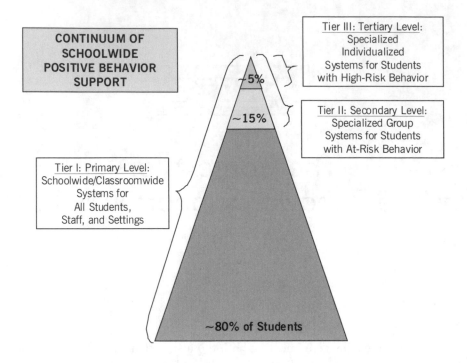

FIGURE 2.1. Three-tiered prevention model for schoolwide positive behavior support. Adapted from Sugai and Horner (2002b). Copyright 2002 by Sage Publications. Adapted by permission.

Tier II interventions. These students may require extra practice in following schoolwide expectations due to poor peer relations, low academic achievement, chaotic home environments, or a multitude of other reasons. *Interventions at the Tier II level are very efficient "packaged" interventions that can be implemented with a group of students needing similar levels of support* (Hawken, Adolphson, MacLeod, & Schumann, 2009; Hawken & Horner, 2003; March & Horner, 2002). The BEP, described in this book, is one example of such an intervention.

Some students will need more support than the BEP can provide. The top part of the triangle represents the approximately 5% of students who engage in the most severe forms of problem behavior and thus require intensive, individualized interventions. For these students, an FBA is conducted and this information is used to develop an individualized behavior support plan (see Crone & Horner, 2003).

COMMITMENT TO PREVENTION OF PROBLEM BEHAVIOR

Schools across the country that have implemented effective schoolwide PBS plans have experienced significant reductions in problem behavior and improvements in the overall climate of their school (Sugai & Horner, 2002a). As a next step, schools should focus on students who engage in frequent problem behavior despite effective schoolwide prevention efforts.

Consider the student who does not have a history of problem behavior. She begins acting out at school when her parents go through a difficult divorce. She could benefit from extra attention or support at school. In some schools, this student's behavior change might be overlooked because it is not severe enough to warrant a behavior support team meeting or to involve the support of special education services. In a school with a BEP intervention in place, a teacher, parent, or other school staff member could inform the BEP team that this student needs additional adult monitoring, feedback, and attention. Within 3–5 school days, the student could be receiving the support she needs. In a school without a BEP intervention, the student's problematic behavior might have to become intense or chronic before she receives support. *By implementing a BEP intervention, schools are committed to preventing problem behavior. In essence, the school is reaching a student before he or she is in crisis and before the student develops a long history of engaging in problem behavior.*

KEY FEATURES AND EXAMPLES OF INTERVENTIONS AT THE TIER II LEVEL

Although the BEP has been shown to be an effective intervention for students with frequent problem behavior (e.g., Filter et al., 2007; Hawken & Horner, 2003), schools should have available a menu of Tier II interventions for responding to the diverse range of student needs. In order to be effective in preventing severe problem behavior, Tier II interventions should contain certain features that differentiate them from Tier I and Tier III levels of behavior support (Hawken & Horner, 2003; March & Horner, 2002). The following key features of Tier II interventions have been outlined by the Office of Special Education Programs (OSEP), Technical Assistance Center on Positive Behavior Intervention and Supports (OSEP, 2005): (1) similar implementation across students (i.e., low effort by teachers); (2) continuous availability and quick access to the intervention; (3) all staff are trained on how to make a referral, and if appropriate how to implement the intervention; (4) intervention is consistent with schoolwide expectations; (5) intervention is flexible based on functional assessment; and (6) data are used continuously to monitor progress on the intervention. These features are listed in Table 2.1 and discussed in further detail below.

The goal of Tier II interventions is to support the approximately 15% of the student population who are at risk but not currently engaging in severe problem behavior (Walker & Horner, 1996). In a school of 500 students, this could include as many as 75 students who need more

TABLE 2.1. Key Features of Tier II Interventions

- Similar implementation across students.
- Continuous availability and quick access to the intervention.
- All school staff are trained on the intervention.
- Intervention is consistent with schoolwide expectations.
- Intervention is flexible based on functional assessment.
- Data are used continuously to monitor progress on the intervention.

support than a schoolwide PBS plan can provide. For this reason, Tier II interventions need to be efficient in terms of time and resources as schools do not have time to implement individualized interventions with all of the students who are at risk. Tier II interventions should involve using a similar set of procedures across a group of students. For example, if social skills training is required for students who have problems with anger management, a similar curriculum should be used across a group of students. If several students are having difficulty with tardies and attendance, Tier II procedures can be designed to more specifically target those problem behaviors.

To be effective in preventing problem behavior, students must be able to access Tier II interventions need to be accessed quickly by students. Unlike more intensive and individualized interventions, which may take weeks of assessment prior to developing a comprehensive behavior intervention plan, Tier II interventions should be accessed by the student relatively quickly—usually within a week (OSEP, 2005). Students are identified quickly and proactively, either by frequently assessing risk factors such as the number of office discipline referrals (ODRs), absences, tardies, or by teacher nomination or referral (Cheney, Blum, & Walker, 2004; Crone, Horner, & Hawken, 2004).

For Tier II interventions that are implemented schoolwide, all staff should receive training on their role in the intervention. The intervention should be consistent with schoolwide expectations (OSEP, 2005). For example, if a middle school has the following schoolwide rules: Be Safe, Be Respectful, Be Responsible, and Hands and Feet to Self, the Tier II intervention should provide more practice and feedback on how to meet these behavioral expectations. Often, these interventions are implemented with the support of a school psychologist, counselor, or paraprofessional, so that the burden of the intervention is not solely on the student's teacher (Crone et al., 2004; Hawken, 2006; Lane et al., 2003). Typically, consultation from experts outside of the school is not necessary or is minimized because the intervention procedures are systematic and standardized (OSEP, 2005).

Tier II interventions should have systems in place to monitor student progress, make modifications, and gradually decrease supports as student behavior improves. One component of this system is a team, which may already exist, such as a student study team (SST) or a more individualized team consisting of teachers, counselors, parents, and students (Christenson, Sinclair, Lehr, & Hurley, 2000). Teams should meet regularly and have systematic procedures for monitoring, troubleshooting, and adding or removing students to or from the intervention (Crone et al., 2004). Team decisions and monitoring of student progress are based on data from a number of different sources depending on the type of program. The team may review student progress on the intervention using information such as the percentage of daily points earned, grades, attendance, participation in school activities, and other indicators of student progress (Crone et al., 2004; Sinclair, Christensen, Evelo, & Hurley, 1998).

Although many of the Tier II interventions have the features described above, not all of the interventions meet all of the OSEP-recommended features. Implementation features of Tier II interventions will vary depending on the needs of individual schools and students. For example, Tier II interventions in elementary schools may focus on preventing escalation of disruptive behavior in the classroom, whereas interventions in large urban high schools may focus on a dropout prevention program (Osher, Dwyer, & Jackson, 2004). Examples of Tier II interventions for social behavior include small-group social skills training (e.g., Lane et al., 2003;

Powers, 2003), mentoring programs such as Check and Connect (Sinclair et al., 1998), new-comer clubs (e.g., programs to teach schoolwide rules/expectations to students who are new and transfer into the school midyear), and systems/programs for supporting students who struggle in unstructured settings (e.g., having a structured recess for a group of students engaging in problem behavior on the playground). Additional Tier II intervention programs include First Steps to Success (Walker et al., 1998), a prevention program for kindergartners with social and behavior problems.

ADVANTAGES OF THE BEP AS A TIER II INTERVENTION

Although each school should have several options for Tier II interventions, in our experience the BEP is an easily implemented and effective Tier II intervention. There are several advantages to implementing the BEP over other types of Tier II interventions. To begin with, depending on school size and resources, up to 30 students can be supported at one time. The students check in with a paraprofessional (e.g., teacher's aide) in the morning. Use of a paraprofessional, rather than a school psychologist or behavioral specialist, has the advantage of reducing the overall costs of delivering the intervention. Many small-group social skills programs can be delivered by trained paraprofessionals, but group sizes typically are limited to five to seven students. Furthermore, when delivering social skills groups, it is difficult to regularly add new members once the groups are formed, and as a result, the intervention can no longer be continuously available for all students. Other Tier II interventions have been shown to be highly effective in reducing problem behavior such as the First Steps to Success intervention (Walker et al., 1998). However, that intervention requires an outside expert to facilitate the intervention and at least 20–40 hours of consultation both with the school and at home. In many cases, this would be cost-prohibitive for schools to implement.

Another major advantage of the BEP is that there is a built-in progress monitoring component. Students receive feedback throughout the day on a Daily Progress Report (DPR) and the percentage of points earned is calculated for each student at the end of each day. This allows teachers and school personnel to easily track daily social behavior and determine if the intervention is working or not for that student. Many Tier II interventions do not have built-in progress monitoring mechanisms. For example, much of the data gathered and published for small-group social skills training is for research purposes, rather than data that is easily collected and readily accessed by school personnel. Tier II interventions such as mentoring often have no ongoing data collection systems, but rather collect data at the end of a certain period of time, such as after 12–16 weeks, to determine the impact of the intervention. To be most effective in preventing serious problem behavior, Tier II interventions need to incorporate ongoing data collection and decision making.

A final advantage is the ease of generalizing the procedures from one student to another. Once teachers have implemented the intervention with one student, they can easily implement the intervention with other students. Teachers rapidly become fluent with implementing the intervention because intervention procedures are the same across students. Teachers learn how to embed the intervention into their classroom schedule and routines so that when a new student begins the intervention, they know how to make it work in their classrooms.

IS THERE RESEARCH THAT SUPPORTS
THE FEASIBILITY AND EFFECTIVENESS OF THE BEP?

Yes, research results support both the ability of schools to adopt and implement the BEP and its effectiveness in reducing problem behavior. The BEP intervention is based on empirically driven behavioral principles for behavior change. Numerous publications (Chafouleas, Christ, Riley-Tillman, Briesch, & Chanese, 2007; Chafouleas, Riley-Tillman, Sassu, LaFrance, & Patwa, 2007; Davies & McLaughlin, 1989; Dougherty & Dougherty, 1977; Leach & Byrne, 1986; Warberg, George, Brown, Chauran, & Taylor-Greene, 1995) support the basic underling principles of the BEP:

1. Define behavioral expectations.
2. Teach the expectations.
3. Provide frequent feedback and reinforcement.
4. Build a regular cycle of checking in and checking out with adults.
5. Formalize consequences for problem behaviors across the school and at home.
6. Use points on DPRs to evaluate intervention effectiveness.

The technology of embedding the BEP into a schoolwide system of behavior support was originally demonstrated at Fern Ridge Middle School (FRMS) in Veneta, Oregon. The leadership staff at FRMS were responsible for developing and testing the original critical features of the BEP. For over 10 years, FRMS has been successfully implementing the BEP. Since its inception, much research has been conducted in both elementary and middle school settings. For example, March and Horner (2002) examined the effects of the BEP on reducing rates of ODRs with middle school students. Using a quasi-experimental design, March and Horner examined the number of ODRs per student both prior to and following BEP implementation. The researchers found that 50% of the students who participated in the BEP intervention had reductions in ODRs following implementation. For the students who were unsuccessful with the BEP, conducting an FBA and implementing an individualized behavior support plan led to significant reductions in problem behavior. Another study with middle school students found that 70% of the students had reductions in ODRs following BEP implementation (Hawken, 2006).

Research on the BEP with elementary school students has demonstrated similar effects. Filter et al. (2007) and Hawken, MacLeod, and Rawlings (2007) found that the BEP was effective in reducing ODRs with 67% and 75%, respectively, of the students who received the intervention. Similar results were found in a study by McCurdy, Kunsch, and Reibstein (2007) in an urban elementary school. In a study by Fairbanks, Sugai, Guardino, and Lathrop (2007), the percentage of students who responded to the BEP was lower (i.e., 40%) than in the Filter et al. (2007) and the Hawken et al. (2007) studies. However, the Fairbanks et al. sample was limited to two second-grade classrooms, rather than examining the BEP schoolwide, as is typically recommended (Crone et al., 2004).

To gain better insight into how the BEP affects problem behavior in the classroom, Hawken and Horner (2003) examined the effects of the BEP on problem behavior and academic engagement using direct observation. Using a multiple baseline design across students, the authors documented reductions in problem behavior in the classroom and increases in academic engagement. These researchers also documented the social acceptability of the intervention. The majority of teachers, parents, and students rated the BEP as (1) helpful in reducing problem behavior, (2) easy to participate in, and (3) worth the time and effort. This study was replicated with four elementary school students by Todd, Kaufman, Meyer, and Horner (2008) with similar results, including reductions in problem behavior as measured by direct observation and rating scales and high levels of social acceptability of the BEP intervention.

Of critical importance when implementing any intervention is the extent to which the intervention can be implemented as planned. All of the aforementioned studies have reported high fidelity of implementation as well as high levels of social acceptability (Fairbanks et al., 2007; Filter et al., 2007; Hawken, 2006; Hawken & Horner, 2003; Hawken, MacLeod, & Rawlings, 2007; March & Horner, 2002). Most importantly, research has documented that implementing the BEP reduces the number of students who require intensive Tier III-level supports (Hawken et al., 2007).

Collectively, these studies have demonstrated the following outcomes:

1. Typical schools are able to implement the BEP successfully.
2. Use of the BEP is functionally related to reduced levels of problem behavior, and, for some students, increased levels of academic engagement.
3. The BEP is likely to be effective with 60–75% of at-risk students.
4. Students who do not find adult attention rewarding appear least likely to respond successfully to the BEP.
5. If a student is not successful on the BEP, conducting an FBA and using the FBA information to adapt the BEP support can be effective in improving behavioral outcomes.

RESOURCES

Building Tier I (Schoolwide) Systems of Behavior Support

Colvin, G., Kameenui, E. J., & Sugai, G. (1993). School-wide and classroom management: Reconceptualizing the integration and management of students with behavior problems in general education. *Education and Treatment of Children, 16,* 361–381.

Colvin, G., Sugai, G., Good, R. H. III, & Lee, Y. (1997). Using active supervision and precorrection to improve transition behaviors in an elementary school. *School Psychology Quarterly, 12,* 344–363.

Lewis, T. J., & Sugai, G. (1999). Effective behavior support: A systems approach to proactive schoolwide management. *Focus on Exceptional Children, 31*(6), 1–24.

Lewis-Palmer, T., Sugai, G., & Larson, S. (1999). Using data to guide decisions about program implementation and effectiveness. *Effective School Practices, 17*(4), 47–53.

Sailor, W., Dunlap, G., Sugai, G., & Horner, R. H. (Eds.). (2009). *Handbook of positive behavior support.* New York: Springer.

Taylor-Greene, S., Brown, D., Nelson, L., Longton, J., Gassman, T., Cohen, J., et al. (1997). School-wide behavioral support: Starting the year off right. *Journal of Behavioral Education, 7,* 99–112.

Todd, A. W., Horner, R. H., Sugai, G., & Sprague, J. R. (1999). Effective behavior support: Strengthening schoolwide systems through a team-based approach. *Effective School Practices, 17*(4), 23–27.

Building Tier II Systems of Behavior Support

Beard-Jordan, K., & Sugai, G. (2004). First Step to Success: An early intervention for elementary children at risk for antisocial behavior. *Behavioral Disorders, 29*, 396–409.

Chafouleas, S., Riley-Tillman, C., Sassu, K., LaFrance, M., & Patwa, S. (2007). Daily behavior report cards: An investigation of the consistency of on-task data across raters and methods. *Journal of Positive Behavior Interventions, 9*(1), 30–37.

Christenson, S. L., Sinclair, M. F., Thurlow, M. L., & Evelo, D. (1999). Promoting student engagement with school using the Check & Connect model. *Australian Journal of Guidance and Counselling, 9*(1), 169–184.

Christenson, S. L., & Thurlow, M. L. (2004). School dropouts: Prevention considerations, interventions, and challenges. *Current Directions in Psychological Science, 13*(1), 36–39.

Fairbanks, S., Sugai, G., Guardino, D., & Lathrop, M. (2007). Response to intervention: Examining classroom behavior support in second grade. *Exceptional Children, 73*(3), 288–310.

Filter, K. J., McKenna, M. K., Benedict, E. A., Horner, R. H., Todd, A. W., & Watson, J. (2007). Check-In/Check-Out: A post-hoc evaluation of an efficient, Tier II-level targeted intervention for reducing problem behaviors in schools. *Education and Treatment of Children, 30*(1), 69–84.

Hawken, L. (2006). School psychologists as leaders in the implementation of a targeted intervention: The Behavior Education Program (BEP). *School Psychology Quarterly, 21*, 91–111.

Hawken, L. S., Adolphson, S. L., MacLeod, K. S., & Schumann, J. (2009). Tier II Tier Interventions and Supports. In W. Sailor, G. Sugai, & R. H. Horner (Eds.), *Handbook of positive behavior support* (pp. 394–414). New York: Springer.

Hawken, L. S., MacLeod, K. S., & Rawlings, L. (2007). Effects of the Behavior Education Program (BEP) on problem behavior with elementary school students. *Journal of Positive Behavior Interventions, 9*, 94–101.

Kauffman, A., Todd, A., Meyer, G., & Horner, R. (2008). The effects of a targeted intervention to reduce problem behavior: Elementary school implementation of Check-In/Check-Out. *Journal of Positive Behavior Interventions, 4*, 194–209.

Lane, K. L., Wehby, J., Menzies, H. M., Doukas, G. L., Munton, S. M., & Gregg, R. M. (2003). Social skills instruction for students at risk for antisocial behavior: The effects of small-group instruction. *Behavioral Disorders, 28*, 229–248.

March, R. E., & Horner, R. H. (2002). Feasibility and contributions of functional behavioral assessment in schools. *Journal of Emotional and Behavioral Disorders, 10*, 158–170.

McCurdy, B. L., Kunsch, C., & Reibstein, S. (2007). Secondary prevention in the urban school: Implementing the Behavior Education Program. *Preventing School Failure, 5*(31), 12–19.

Todd, A. W., Kaufman, A., Meyer, G., & Horner, R. H. (2008). The effects of a targeted intervention to reduce problem behaviors: Elementary school implementation of Check-In–Check-Out. *Journal of Positive Behavioral Interventions, 10*, 46–55.

Walker, H. M., Kavanagh, K., Stiller, B., Golly, A., Severson, H. H., & Feil, E. G. (1998). First Step to Success: An early intervention approach for preventing school antisocial behavior. *Journal of Emotional and Behavioral Disorders, 6*(2), 66–80.

Building Tier III Systems of Behavior Support

Benazzi, L., Horner, R. H., & Good, R. H. (2006). Effects of behavior support team composition on the technical adequacy and contextual fit of behavior support plans. *Journal of Special Education, 40*(3), 160–170.

Borgmeier, C., & Horner, R. H. (2006). An evaluation of the predictive validity of confidence ratings in identifying accurate functional behavioral assessment hypothesis statements. *Journal of Positive Behavior Interventions, 8*(2), 100–105.

Crone, D. A., & Horner, R. H. (2003). *Building positive behavior support systems in schools: Functional behavioral assessment.* New York: Guilford Press.

O'Neill, R. E., Horner, R. H., Albin, R. W., Sprague, J. R., Storey, K., & Newton, J. S. (1997). *Functional assessment for problem behavior: A practical handbook* (2nd ed.). Pacific Grove, CA: Brooks/Cole.

Repp, A. C., & Horner, R. H. (Eds.). (1999). *Functional analysis of problem behavior: From effective assessment to effective support.* Belmont, CA: Wadsworth.

CHAPTER 3

The Basic BEP

Critical Features and Processes

DEFINING FEATURES OF THE BEP

The BEP has several critical defining features that establish it as an efficient, effective, and sustainable Tier II intervention. These features include the following:

1. The BEP is an *efficient* system that is capable of providing behavioral support to a moderate-sized group of at-risk students (approximately 10–30 students) at the same time.
2. The BEP is continuously available within the school, so a student who is identified as needing support can get access to the BEP within 3–5 days.
3. The backbone of the BEP involves a daily "check-in" and "check-out" with a respected adult.
4. The BEP is designed to increase the likelihood that each class period begins with a positive interaction with the teacher or supervisor.
5. The BEP increases the frequency of contingent feedback from the teacher or supervisor.
6. The BEP requires low effort from teachers. That is, teachers should experience significant, positive changes in student behavior even though the individual teacher's BEP workload will be minimal.
7. The BEP links behavioral and academic support.
8. The BEP is implemented and supported by all administrators, teachers, and staff in the school building.
9. Students choose to participate and cooperate with the BEP system. They are not required to do so.
10. The BEP employs continuous monitoring of student behavior and active use of data for decision making.

Based on Behavioral Principles

The BEP is a school-based intervention for providing daily support to students at risk for developing serious or chronic behavior problems. The BEP is based on three "big ideas" from behavioral research:

1. At-risk students benefit from (a) clearly defined expectations, (b) frequent feedback, (c) consistency, and (d) positive reinforcement that is contingent on meeting goals.
2. Problem behavior and poor academic performance are often linked.
3. Behavior support begins with the development of effective adult–student relationships.

Implementation of the BEP creates increased collaboration between school and home and increased opportunities for self-management. Each of these is also important for behavioral change by students at risk. The administration and staff at your school will apply these three "big ideas" as they develop your BEP system.

A Brief Tour of BEP Elements

The elements and procedures for implementing the BEP are described in more depth later in this chapter. It is helpful, however, to have a general overview of the key elements.

1. *Personnel.* The BEP program is managed by a BEP coordinator and a behavior support team. All teaching faculty in the school have an opportunity to participate.
2. *Student identification.* A student is identified to enter the BEP in one of three ways: (a) the behavior support team screens student variables associated with risk (e.g., an increase in the rate of ODRs or absences); (b) through systematic screening of all students for behavior problems; and/or (c) by teacher nomination. When a student is nominated for participation, an agreement is developed between the student, the family, and the BEP coordinator, and a BEP plan of support is defined. All students participating in the BEP agree to willingly participate.
3. *Process.* The BEP involves a daily cycle and a weekly (or every 2 weeks) cycle. The daily cycle consists of the following:

   - The student arrives at school and checks in with an adult (e.g., the BEP coordinator). At this check-in, the student receives his or her Daily Progress Report (DPR).
   - The student carries the DPR throughout the day and hands it to the teacher or supervisor at the start of the day (for elementary school) or each class period (for middle or high school).
   - The student retrieves the DPR after each class period and receives feedback from the teacher or supervisor related to expected social behaviors.
   - At the end of the day the student returns the DPR to the BEP coordinator, determines whether daily point goals were met, and carries a copy of the DPR home.
   - Family members receive the DPR, deliver recognition for success, and sign the form. The next morning the student returns the signed DPR to the BEP coordinator.

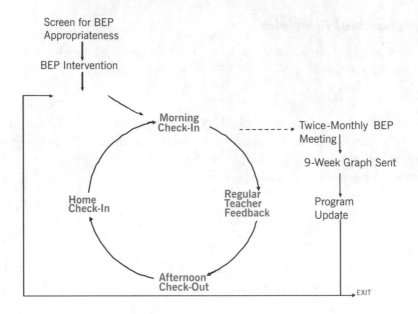

FIGURE 3.1. The BEP intervention cycle.

On a weekly (or every 2 weeks) basis, the behavior support team holds a meeting to review the percentage of points earned by each student and to adjust support options as needed. A diagram of the basic BEP cycle is provided in Figure 3.1.

Antecedent Features of the BEP

Antecedents are events or situations that occur before problem behavior. They can be thought of as the trigger that sets off the behavior. In order to prevent problem behavior, the key is to reduce the likelihood that the behavior will occur by making adjustments to its behavioral triggers.

There are certain antecedent features of the BEP that increase its overall effectiveness. The BEP creates a structure that eliminates antecedents to *problem behavior* by increasing antecedents for *positive* or *appropriate behavior*. These antecedent features include (1) provision of school supplies as needed at the beginning of the school day, (2) a prompt to have a good day, (3) a prompt to have a good class period, and (4) a reminder of behavioral expectations.

Disorganization is a common characteristic of the students on the BEP intervention. These students often come to school without a pen or pencil, or without an adequate supply of paper. Coming unprepared for class is an antecedent, or trigger, for getting into trouble as soon as the teacher gives the class a direction. For the students on the BEP, this entire scenario can be avoided by checking to see if they have paper and a pen first thing in the morning and providing them with whatever materials they are missing before sending them to class. When a student checks in in the morning, the BEP coordinator reminds him or her to have a good day and prompts the student to remember the schoolwide expectations. The BEP coordinator also asks the student what he or she is working on to improve behavior (e.g., "I need to work on keeping my hands and feet to myself"). This daily prompt can mean the difference between starting the day out poorly or making better choices that start the day off in the right direction. Finally, students on the BEP also receive a prompt at the beginning of each class period (for middle and high school students) or at each class transition (for elementary students). This prompt reminds students of the class and school expectations and helps the students keep their behavior on target during class time.

FOR WHOM IS THE BEP MOST APPROPRIATE?

The BEP is most appropriate for students who are considered "at risk" for developing serious or chronic behavior problems. These students consistently have trouble in "low-level" problem areas. For example, they frequently come to school unprepared, talk out, talk back to the teacher, or cause minor disruptions in the classroom. In other words, their behavior is disruptive, detrimental to instruction, and interferes with their own learning and that of others, but is not dangerous or violent. The BEP involves frequent positive interaction between students and teachers as well as increased monitoring of student behavior by adults at school and home. For this reason, the BEP will be most effective for students who engage in problem behavior in order to obtain adult attention or who find adult attention reinforcing. Students who are not reinforced by adult attention, or who even find it aversive, would not be good candidates for the BEP. For those students, the BEP could actually worsen their behavior.

The BEP is not adequate for students who engage in serious or violent behaviors or infractions, such as bringing a weapon to school or vandalizing the school. While those individuals might receive some benefit from the BEP, such students require more individualized attention and support than can be provided by the BEP alone.

The BEP is not necessary for students who have been sent to the office on rare occasions or whose behavior is actually driven by a problem in the environmental setting. For example, school cafeterias can be loud, chaotic places. A student who is repeatedly referred to the office for yelling in the cafeteria is not an immediate candidate for additional behavior support. In a loud, chaotic cafeteria, the setting should be assessed and modified first. If the student's problem behavior continues, and is highly discrepant from the behavior of peers in the same setting, the student might then benefit from the BEP or from individualized behavior support.

When deciding who is appropriate for the BEP system, it is important to remember that the problem behaviors of students eligible for the BEP will look different in elementary school than in middle or high school. A typical BEP student in elementary school might have difficulty taking his or her turn, refuse to share materials with others, have difficulty remaining seated or completing tasks, or be mildly aggressive toward other students, especially on the playground or in areas with a poorer ratio of adult-to-child supervision. A BEP student in middle school may be more likely to use inappropriate language, be frequently late to class, be defiant toward adults, or refuse to do work. *Whether in elementary, middle, or high school, the key is to identify those students who have a consistent pattern of problem behavior that has not yet reached serious or chronic levels.* Table 3.1 provides a summary of the characteristics of good candidates and poor candidates for the BEP.

TABLE 3.1. Appropriate and Inappropriate Candidates for the BEP

Appropriate candidates for the BEP	Inappropriate candidates for the BEP
• Engage in problem behavior throughout the day, in multiple settings.	• Engage in problem behavior during one class period or only in unstructured settings (e.g., playground, hallways, lunchroom, bus area).
• Engage in mild acting-out behaviors such as talking out, off task, or out of seat.	• Engage in serious or violent behavior such as *extreme* noncompliance/defiance, aggression, injury to self or others.
• Problem behavior is not related to trying to escape difficult academic work. Assessments indicate instructional material is at the student's level.	• Problem behavior mainly occurs when student is trying to escape a difficult task or academic subject. Assessments indicate instructional material is not at the student's level.
• Problem behavior is maintained by adult attention and/or the student finds adult attention reinforcing.	• Problem behavior is maintained by escape from academic tasks and/or the student *does not* find adult attention reinforcing.

IDENTIFYING STUDENTS FOR THE BEP

There are several ways students can be identified for the BEP including examining existing student data, systematically screening all students for social behavior problems, and/or teacher referral. Regardless of how students are *identified* for the BEP, determining the *appropriateness* of the BEP for a particular student should be made by the behavior support team.

Examining Existing Student Data

One way to identify students for the BEP is to examine existing data sources that may indicate a student may be at risk. School personnel typically have access to data on the number of student absences, tardies, in-school detentions, and suspensions. Some schools employ, and keep records of, a schoolwide system of interclass time-out for inappropriate behavior, such as Think Time (Nelson, 1997). If the data show that a student is repeatedly sent out of the classroom for behavioral issues, that student is at risk for serious problem behavior and may be a good candidate for the BEP.

Schools that have implemented behavior support (with fidelity) at the Tier I level have systematically defined those problem behaviors that should result in an ODR. These ODR data can be organized and summarized using systems such as the Schoolwide Information System (SWIS; May et al., 2000). Schools that have a systematic process for regularly tracking office discipline referrals are more efficient in identifying students at risk, as these systems allow school personnel to answer questions such as: Who has been referred to the office? How many times? For what problems? Under what circumstances?

If ODRs are systematically tracked and recorded so that it is easy to examine the data, meaningful referral patterns can be readily identified. The school may choose to "red flag" any student who has received a total of two or more ODRs in a month. Depending on the average number of ODRs per student/per month received at a school, the school may choose a higher or lower standard for identifying at-risk students. With a systematic and efficient tracking system, it would be simple to determine which students fall into the "red flag" category.

Our experience tells us that the number of ODRs that indicate risk at one school are different than that at another school, and the threshold for risk depends greatly on the specific student population. For this reason, we cannot specify a criterion number of ODRs that should result in identification for BEP placement. As a general guide, though, students who receive *two to five* ODRs will likely require additional intervention beyond what is provided by the Tier I level of positive behavior support.

A systematic tracking system allows the school to easily determine which students are receiving the most referrals, under what circumstances, and for which types of problem behaviors. This information is critical to identifying those students who need behavioral support. In terms of evaluation, it also allows for a comparison of the student's behavior before and after behavioral support was implemented.

Using Discipline Referral Data: Examples

Figure 3.2 illustrates the number of referrals received by individual students. These sample data are taken from a school of approximately 350 students. Approximately seven students were responsible for almost half of the ODRs processed at that school (students AA, AB, AC, AD, AE, AF, and AG). (Between them, the seven students received 70 ODRs out of 146 total referrals at the school.) These numbers are not unusual. On average, approximately 1–5% of the students in a school will have serious, chronic problem behaviors. These students will need *Tier III* intervention, including intensive assessment and individualized behavior support. These seven students are not the best candidates for a *Tier II* intervention. On the other hand, note the 15 students who received three to five ODRs. These students may be at risk for developing chronic patterns of problem behavior. It is likely that these students would benefit from a Tier II intervention such as the BEP intervention.

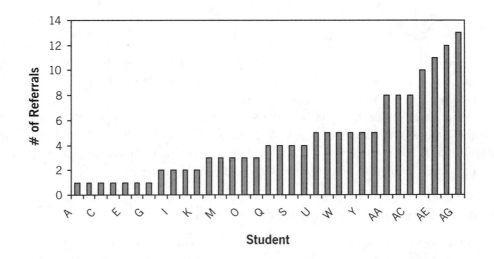

FIGURE 3.2. Referral data by individual students, 2009–2010.

Student Name: Student W

Behavior	Time	Date	Setting	Referral issued by:
Noncompliance	10:45	9/17	Social Studies	Teacher
Disruption	12:50	9/19	Language Arts	Teacher
Inappropriate language	2:20	10/12	Gym/P.E.	Educational assistant
Noncompliance	8:15	10/15	Math	Teacher
Noncompliance	11:00	11/2	Social Studies	Teacher

FIGURE 3.3. Summary of referral data for an individual student.

Figure 3.3 illustrates the referral pattern for an individual student. This student has five ODRs. The figure summarizes the student's referral record. The student received three ODRs for noncompliance, one ODR for disruption, and one ODR for inappropriate language. The student has a consistent pattern of engaging in mildly disruptive and defiant problem behavior. In addition, Figure 3.3 shows the times and places where the behavioral incident occurred and who issued the referral. This particular student has engaged in problem behavior across the school day with a range of staff. This student is a good candidate for the BEP. The BEP will provide behavioral feedback and support across each of the class periods where the student has experienced trouble.

In contrast, the BEP intervention would be less appropriate for a student who received the same number of ODRs if each referral always originated in the same class period or setting. In that case, it is more likely that the student's behavior can be improved by modifying that specific routine or setting associated with the ODRs. This is an example of trying to leverage your intervention to get the biggest impact for the least amount of effort. If all of a student's ODRs originate in unstructured settings such as the hallway, lunchroom, or cafeteria, the BEP is not the best intervention. Because the BEP is mainly a classroom intervention, it will not be as effective in unstructured settings.

Teacher or Parent Referral

Teachers can also make referrals to the BEP. Teachers requesting support from a behavior support team should provide data (e.g., behavior logs, interclass time-out data), that documents that the student is engaging in repetitive problem behavior. The behavior support team then examines the teacher's data as well as ODRs, absences, tardies, and academic performance data. Although it is rare, parents can also make a referral to the BEP. It will be important for the behavior support team to determine if the student is engaging in behaviors that indicate he or she would benefit from, and be an appropriate candidate for, the BEP.

Systematic Screening for Behavior Problems

While some students are easily identified for the BEP using teacher referral or ODRs, other students engage in internalizing behaviors (e.g., depression, anxiety, withdrawal), requiring more comprehensive assessment in order to be identified. While students with internalizing behaviors cause less disruption to the learning environment, these students are equally in need of appropriate interventions. For students who engage in internalizing behaviors or who present less intensive externalizing behaviors, office ODRs may not provide adequate information. For these students, other effective screening tools are necessary to proactively identify at-risk students before these students require interventions at the Tier III level.

Some schools implement systematic screening tools for early identification of at-risk students. The Systematic Screening for Behavior Disorders rating system (SSBD; Walker & Severson, 1992), for example, allows identification of students who may benefit from Tier II interventions such as the BEP (e.g., Cheney et al., 2004). The SSBD is a multiple-stage approach, implemented schoolwide, to identify students at risk. The first stage involves teachers identifying students in their classrooms who are at high risk for externalizing and internalizing disorders. In the second stage, teachers complete behavior rating scales on the identified students to determine if further assessment should occur. The third stage involves direct observation in the classroom for students who pass through stages 1 and 2 and who appear to be most at risk.

A second screening measure that can be used to identify students for Tier II interventions is the Social Skills Rating Scale (SSRS; Gresham & Elliot, 1990). The SSRS is a set of three norm-referenced rating scales that allow schools to combine teacher, parent, and student reports to gain a more complete understanding of a students' social behavior. The SSRS, in combination with the *Social Skills Intervention Guide: Practical Strategies for Social Skills Training* (Elliot & Gresham, 1991) can be useful in helping schools identify which students need additional intervention.

Although systematic screening of all students may be more time-consuming, recent research indicates that screening tools such as the SSBD and other teacher nomination strategies might be more accurate mechanisms than ODR counts in identifying students who are at risk, particularly for students who engage in internalizing problem behaviors (Blum, 2006; Kincaid, 2007).

HOW IS THE BEP INTERVENTION INTEGRATED INTO A SCHOOL'S OTHER IDENTIFICATION SYSTEMS FOR STUDENTS IN NEED?

Every school provides a range of services to students with diverse needs. For example, every public school provides Title I and special education services. Many schools provide mentoring programs, extracurricular tutoring, or even mental health services. Each service typically requires a process for identifying students who are eligible for, or in need of, the service. The more services available, the more cumbersome it may be to navigate the multiple identification processes. Adding the BEP intervention can further complicate matters.

School administrators should carefully coordinate the multiple services offered within their school. Each school should examine the identification processes used for each service and assess if any of the interventions are inefficient, redundant, or overly bureaucratic. Representatives from each service area (e.g., BEP coordinator, special education teacher, and school nurse) should meet. They should determine how to reduce any inefficiency, redundancy, or red tape created by their multiple services.

The first step is to build awareness of the services that are provided by each professional or team. The next step is to build collaboration or partnership among the various services. Real collaboration among service providers in a school will reduce the likelihood that services provided by one group will be replicated or even contraindicated by another group.

The teams used (or created) to develop and implement the BEP will vary from school to school. In some schools, the schoolwide behavior support team designs the BEP to fit the culture of their school, but a multidisciplinary team or teacher assistance team is in charge of examining data for decision making. In other schools, a multidisciplinary team that is in charge of both academic and behavior support embeds the BEP implementation and evaluation into their existing meetings.

We recommend that schools review their current set of teams and consider if a team already exists that can manage BEP implementation. Some schools find it helpful to list the teams/committees at a school, along with the purpose of the committee and the staff involved. The "Working Smarter, Not Harder" sample graphic illustrated in Figure 3.4 can be used as an organizing structure for accomplishing this task. (A blank organizer is included as a handout in Appendix B.1.)

DECISION PROCESS FOR BEP PLACEMENT

Before a student can be placed on the BEP, the behavior support team must determine that the student is an appropriate candidate for the intervention.

Referral Form

Each school should have a referral or request for assistance form that is used to access the behavior support team. An example of such a form is included in Appendix B.2. The referral form should include the student's name, the date, the name of the referring person, the reason for referral (i.e., description of problem[s]), the hypothesized reason for why the problem is occurring (i.e., What does the student gain by misbehaving? What skills is he or she missing?), and the strategies tried thus far. There should be a place on the form to summarize relevant academic data (e.g., Oral Reading Fluency scores) and behavior data (e.g., number of absences, tardies, interclass time-outs). All the faculty and staff within a building should be familiar with how to use the form to make a referral to the behavior support team. The referral forms should be easily accessible and, once completed, should be given to the person in charge of the behavior support team.

BEP Placement Decision

As discussed previously, not all students who are referred for the BEP will be appropriate for it. School staff should also recognize that some students may have behavior that is so chronic or severe that it cannot be remedied by a simple intervention like the BEP. These students will require more intensive, individualized behavior support (Crone & Horner, 2003).

Once a referral is received, the behavior support team will decide if a student should be placed on the BEP. If the student is an appropriate candidate, the behavior support team should secure parental/guardian consent for the intervention. (See Appendix B.3 for a sample copy of a parental permission form.)

Committee, project, or initiative	Purpose	Outcome	Target group	Staff involved
Behavior support team	Address students who are engaging in problem behavior	Provide teachers with interventions	Students with repetitive behavior problems	School psychologist, principal, representative sample of staff
Schoolwide climate committee	Improve school climate	Reduce behavior referrals, increase safety, increase organization and understanding of school routines	All students and staff	Principal, counselor, teachers, educational assistants
Discipline team	Provide negative consequences for inappropriate behavior	Individual students receive disciplinary action as necessary	Students with office discipline referrals	Vice principal, counselor
School spirit committee	Increase school spirit and bonding to school	Organize pep assemblies, appreciation events, and other activities	All students	Interested teachers and staff
After-school tutoring programs	Provide opportunity for help with homework and other tutoring needs	Students receive small-group instruction in academic areas of need	Students with specific academic needs	School counselor and interested teachers and staff

FIGURE 3.4. Example of a completed Working Smarter, Not Harder organizer.

Gathering Baseline Data and Signing Contracts

A powerful way to test the effectiveness of the BEP intervention for an individual student is to begin by collecting 3–5 days of baseline data. Baseline data can be collected during the time period that the team is waiting for parents to provide consent for participation. Baseline data is gathered by having the teacher rate the student's behavior on the DPR, but not provide verbal feedback to the student. The behavior support team provides the teacher with a packet of three to five DPRs. During the baseline period, the student should not be aware that his or her behavior is being rated. Students do not check in or check out with the BEP coordinator during this time period.

Baseline data can help establish if a student truly needs the intervention. It can also be used to determine the daily point goals for the student. Moreover, baseline data provide a gauge for assessing a teacher's commitment to implementing the intervention. If the teacher is unwilling or sporadic in completing baseline DPRs, it is unlikely that he or she will follow through with the feedback, reinforcement, and other critical components of the BEP intervention. For middle and high school settings, teachers for each class period should be given DPRs and the BEP coordinator should gather and summarize the baseline data.

Once consent for participation is obtained from the parent or guardian, it is recommended that the parents/guardians and student sign a "contract" delineating each person's role in BEP implementation. In some schools, one document serves as both the parental contract and the parental permission form.

BEP IMPLEMENTATION

In this book, we present a basic BEP process as well as ways to adapt the intervention to meet specific needs. Adaptations and elaborations on the basic BEP are described in detail in Chapter 8. Typically, students are placed on the basic BEP program if they have attention-motivated problem behavior and/or if they find adult attention reinforcing. In some cases, the basic BEP may prove to be ineffective or inadequate for a particular student, and the behavior support team should consider introducing modifications after a few weeks of implementation. Figure 3.5 presents a decision tree for deciding whether or not a student should participate in the BEP system and the type of modifications to the basic BEP that may be required. Modifications to the basic BEP are discussed more fully in Chapter 8.

The following section outlines the *basic* BEP process for an elementary and a middle school student. Information on how this basic BEP can be adapted for high school is presented in Chapter 9 and preschool modifications are presented in Chapter 10.

BASIC BEP CYCLES

There are critical features of the BEP process that must occur on a daily, weekly (or twice-monthly), and quarterly basis. The daily features involve both the daily participation of the identified students and the day-to-day management and implementation of the system. On a weekly or twice-monthly basis the data should be summarized, reviewed, and used in making

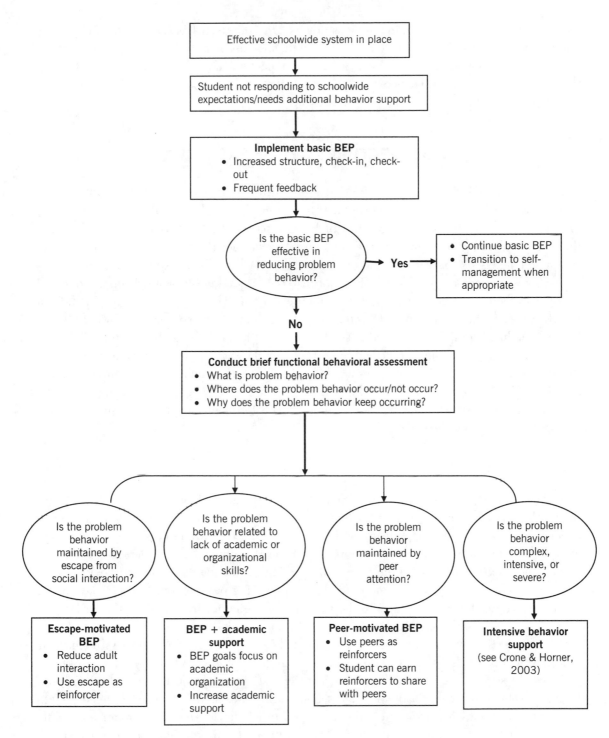

FIGURE 3.5. Decision tree for BEP placement.

data-based decisions regarding individual students. On a quarterly basis, there should be a system for providing feedback to the teachers and staff, students, and parents on the impact of the BEP. Feedback should include a discussion of the impact for individual students as well as for the overall school climate. This next section details the critical features necessary at each point in this process.

DAILY FEATURES OF THE BASIC BEP

Each student on the BEP starts and ends each day with a positive contact with an adult in the school and receives frequent monitoring and behavioral feedback throughout the day. In the morning, the students check in with the BEP coordinator. The BEP coordinator makes sure that each student has brought all of the necessary materials for the day (e.g., pencil, paper, and assignment notebook) and reminds the student to follow the schoolwide expectations. In elementary schools, it is not as important to check for materials as students typically keep these school supplies in their desks or somewhere else in their classroom. The student picks up a DPR from the BEP coordinator and begins the school day. In each class, the student checks in with the teacher and hands him or her the DPR. The teacher uses the DPR to rate the student's behavior within that class period (for middle and high school) or class activity (for elementary school). In this manner, the student receives continual behavioral feedback and prompting throughout the school day. The DPR is turned in to the BEP coordinator at the end of the day. A copy of the DPR is sent home for the student's parents or guardians to review and sign—a simple strategy for including daily home–school collaboration.

Middle School

Schools should identify a team to support BEP implementation. Due to personnel shortages, some schools have relied on one individual to coordinate the entire BEP intervention. In our experience, schools that adopt a team model to support the BEP are more successful at implementing and maintaining the intervention than schools that depend on one person to build and sustain the program. Similar to the process of working with students requiring special education services, a team approach is more effective in assessing progress on the BEP, developing recommendations for modifications to the BEP, and planning for transition off the BEP intervention. Throughout this chapter, we assume that a team model is adopted.

It is easiest to illustrate the BEP by describing the entire process for a sample student. Our sample student is called Jeremy. Jeremy is a seventh-grade student. He received seven ODRs the previous school year and two ODRs during the first few weeks of the current school year. Jeremy's referral summary for the previous school year is presented in Figure 3.6. According to his summary, Jeremy has a pattern of disruptive, off-task behavior in the classroom and mildly aggressive behavior toward peers. The majority of his problem behaviors occur in classroom settings. According to his teachers, problem behavior is more prevalent toward the end of the class period.

The behavior support team decides that Jeremy would be a good candidate for the BEP. Three requirements must be met prior to implementation of the BEP. First, baseline data must be gathered by his teachers. Second, the BEP coordinator must obtain permission from Jeremy's

Student Name: Jeremy Walker

Behavior	Time	Date	Location	Referral issued by:
Fighting	2:00	9/23	Gym	Gym teacher
Inappropriate language	8:30	10/12	Room 214	Homeroom teacher
Disruption/noncompliance	1:15	11/6	Art room	Art teacher
Inappropriate language	12:00	12/15	Room 226	Science teacher
Disruption/noncompliance	10:15	1/17	Music room	Music teacher
Fighting	9:00	2/15	Hallway	Assistant principal
Fighting	11:00	3/03	Room 124	LA teacher

FIGURE 3.6. Summary of referral data for Jeremy.

parents. Third, the purpose and process of the BEP must be explained to both Jeremy and his parents, and they must agree to actively participate.

The BEP coordinator and school counselor arrange a meeting with Jeremy's parents during the school day. Both parents agree that the BEP would be a positive support for Jeremy. They are eager to have him begin and are willing to cooperate and participate. While his parents are still at the school, Jeremy is excused from his classroom to attend the meeting. At this point, a detailed explanation of the BEP intervention is presented to Jeremy and his parents and baseline data is shared.

Jeremy's baseline data shows that he is meeting behavioral expectations 50–60% of the time. It is likely that he would benefit from the additional feedback and reinforcement provided by the BEP. During the meeting, the roles and responsibilities of each participant—Jeremy, his parents, and the school—are discussed. The BEP coordinator provides Jeremy with training on where to check in/check out, how to request feedback from teachers, and other critical components of the basic BEP. (For more detailed information on BEP training for students, refer to Chapter 5.) Finally, a daily point goal for Jeremy is agreed upon.

The goal for most students on the BEP is to receive 80% of the total points per day. Given that Jeremy averaged 50–60% of daily points during the baseline period (without feedback or reinforcement), 80% of daily points is considered a realistic goal. It is important that the initial point goal is set at a level that the student can reasonably achieve. The student must experience success with the BEP at the initiation of the intervention or his commitment and interest in the program will rapidly dissolve. For some students to be successful on the BEP, a lower initial point goal (e.g., 60% of the total points) may be necessary. The point goal can be increased as the student demonstrates success. Baseline data will help you determine which goals are realistic.

At the end of Jeremy's meeting, everyone is given an opportunity to ask any remaining questions and they are answered. Jeremy begins the BEP the following day.

The school day begins at 8:30 in the morning. Students can complete the BEP check-in between 8:00 and 8:30. At 8:00 A.M., the BEP coordinator opens the doors to the counseling office, and the BEP students begin to arrive. Because the students view the BEP as positive support, not punishment, many bring their friends to morning check-in. (Some friends even ask if they can be put on the BEP intervention!) The students who have been on the BEP system for a week or more are familiar with the routine. Morning check-in usually proceeds smoothly and efficiently because the routine is so predictable.

Jeremy arrives on time the first morning and is greeted by the BEP coordinator, one of the school's educational assistants (i.e., paraprofessional). She commends Jeremy for remembering where and when to show up. Every day, each student picks up a new DPR. Jeremy takes a DPR. The cards are printed on duplicate paper so that one copy can go home to his parents to sign, while the original copy is kept for school records. An example of Jeremy's DPR is presented in Figure 3.7. (A blank version of this form is included in Appendix B.4 and a second example of a middle school DPR is included in Appendix B.5.)

This middle school has a block schedule with "A" days (first, second, third, homeroom, and fourth period) and "B" days (fifth, sixth, seventh, homeroom, and eighth period). For schools that do not have block schedules, all periods should be given a separate column on the DPR. Before leaving the check-in room, Jeremy puts his name and the date on the card. Next, the BEP coordinator checks to make sure that Jeremy has all of the materials he will need for the day. Jeremy opens his backpack to show her that he has loose-leaf paper, a pencil, a pen, and his assignment notebook/planner. If students arrive in the morning without all of their necessary materials, the BEP coordinator provides them with a few sheets of paper or pencils and pens, as needed. Students are reminded and encouraged to come to school prepared the next day. After Jeremy has completed check-in, he is sent off with a prompt to have a good day and to follow the rules listed on his DPR.

Often, the students are given "Thumbs Up!" tickets for checking in responsibly and being prepared with their materials. Thumbs Up! tickets are part of a token economy system set up by the school to encourage support of the five schoolwide expectations. All students in the building have the opportunity to earn Thumbs Up! tickets throughout the day for demonstrating appropriate behavior. A sample Thumbs Up! ticket is illustrated in Figure 3.8. (A blank version can be found in Appendix B.6.)

Once Jeremy leaves check-in, he has a few minutes before school starts. At the beginning of each class period, Jeremy gives the DPR to his teacher. All of the teachers in the school have participated in an inservice on the BEP, so each teacher knows how to respond to Jeremy's entry into each period. When a student brings a DPR to a teacher, it serves as an opportunity for the teacher to offer a brief positive comment or prepare the student for the class. Often this is the time when teachers will remind students of behaviors they are working on, for example "Yesterday you had a difficult time completing your work. Let's just try harder today." It is recommended that teachers keep the DPRs on their desk to prompt them to provide feedback at the end of the period versus placing the DPR on the student's desk. At the end of the class period, the teacher rates Jeremy on a scale of 0–2 for how well he did for each behavioral expectation. A "2" means "Yes"; the student met the behavioral goal. A "1" means the student did "So-so," and a "0" means "No," the student did not meet that goal for that class period. Jeremy gives his DPR to each teacher throughout the day.

Teachers are encouraged to explain their choice of ratings to the students and to praise them on days when they meet or come close to meeting their behavioral goals (receive 2's on a majority of the goals). Teachers are also encouraged to hand out Thumbs Up! tickets to students who meet all of the behavioral goals in one class period. In this way, the BEP student receives continual feedback and prompting and frequent reinforcement for appropriate behavior. In

Daily Progress Report—Middle School, Example 1

(A- Day)   B-Day

Name: _Jeremy Walker_   Date: _11/18_

Teachers: Please indicate YES (2), So-So (1), or No (0) regarding the student's achievement for the following goals.

Goals	1/5	2/6	3/7	HR	4/8
Be respectful	~~2~~ 1 0	2 ~~1~~ 0	~~2~~ 1 0	~~2~~ 1 0	2 ~~1~~ 0
Be responsible	~~2~~ 1 0	2 ~~1~~ 0	~~2~~ 1 0	~~2~~ 1 0	~~2~~ 1 0
Keep hands and feet to self	2 ~~1~~ 0	~~2~~ 1 0	2 1 ~~0~~	~~2~~ 1 0	2 ~~1~~ 0
Follow directions	2 ~~1~~ 0	~~2~~ 1 0	2 ~~1~~ 0	~~2~~ 1 0	~~2~~ 1 0
Be there— be ready	~~2~~ 1 0	~~2~~ 1 0	~~2~~ 1 0	~~2~~ 1 0	~~2~~ 1 0
TOTAL POINTS	8	8	7	10	8
TEACHER INITIALS	A.K.	B.D.	R.S.	J.T.	B.L.

BEP Daily Goal   _40/ 50_   BEP Daily Score   _41/ 50_

In training _____   BEP Member _X___   _Jeremy Walker_
                                                       Student signature

Teacher comments: Please state briefly any specific behaviors or achievements that demonstrate the student's progress. (If additional space is required, please attach a note and indicate so below.)

Period 1/5 _Behavior is improving!_

Period 2/6 _____

Period 3/7 _____

Homeroom _Excellent behavior today!_

Period 4/8 _____

Parent/Caregiver Signature: _Angel Walker_

Parent/Caregiver Comments: _Keep up the good work!_

FIGURE 3.7. Jeremy's completed DPR.

```
                         THUMBS UP! TICKET

      Student name:     Jeremy
      Issued by:        Teacher
      Date:             9/17

                         WAY TO GO!
```

FIGURE 3.8. Example of a completed Thumbs Up! ticket for Jeremy.

addition, doing poorly in one class does not ruin the rest of the day. Each class period is a clean slate—a new chance to meet behavioral goals.

At the end of the day, Jeremy returns his DPR to the BEP coordinator. Both check-in and check-out are in the same location, so the routine is predictable. The BEP coordinator keeps the top copy and sends the second copy home with Jeremy for his parents. Check-out goes quickly, as many students have to get on the bus. However, it provides another opportunity for a positive adult contact. It also provides an opportunity to prompt Jeremy again for appropriate behavior. In this school, if students have met their goal for the day, they are allowed to select a small snack (candy, juice, crackers, etc.) to take with them. Other schools have different reinforcement systems. You should design one to fit your school (see Chapter 6 for suggestions on designing reinforcement systems).

Jeremy is expected to give the copy of his DPR to his parents. If he does not give it to them, they are expected to ask for it. There is a place for the parents to make positive comments on the DPR, sign it, and send it back. Jeremy returns the copy of the DPR to the BEP coordinator the next morning at check-in. This is a very simple way to increase the communication and collaboration between home and school—something that is always critical, but especially so during the middle school years.

One of the BEP coordinator's responsibilities is to enter the daily BEP data into a database. It is critical that the school reserve enough time each week for the BEP coordinator to accomplish this task. The BEP coordinator collects the daily BEP data and enters the *percentage* of points (*not* total number of points) earned into a database for all of the BEP students. This should be done at least on a weekly basis, if not a daily basis, or it is easy to fall behind.

The daily percentage point data can be graphed to illustrate each individual student's progress on the BEP. Students are typically held to a goal criterion of 80% of total possible points. For example, if 50 points are possible throughout the day, students have met their goal if they have received 40 or more points. Students who fall below this criterion have not met their goal. If a student goes for several days without meeting his or her goal, or if the student's performance is highly variable, the behavior support team should see this as a red flag and should investigate, possibly modifying the intervention or increasing support for a particular student.

Figure 3.9 illustrates Jeremy's BEP data for the first week, as well as his data from baseline. It appears that Jeremy struggled in the beginning of the week, but by Thursday he had begun to meet his goal of 80% of points. From this data, the behavior support team might conclude that Jeremy is beginning to adjust to the BEP intervention and that he has the potential to benefit

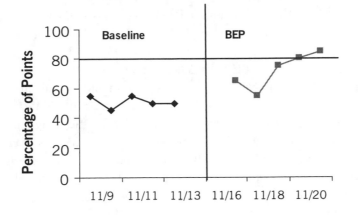

FIGURE 3.9. Jeremy's BEP data for the first week.

from it. The team will continue to monitor and examine his daily data for patterns of behavioral success or struggle.

Elementary School

For students in elementary school, the BEP process is quite similar, but the DPR differs. The DPR reflects natural transitions of elementary school classrooms (such as the transition between reading and math) versus changes in class periods for middle and high school students. The behavioral goals need to be written in a manner that is understandable for younger students. The younger students may require visuals (e.g., smiley faces, thumbs-up picture) to make it clear when goals are met and not met. (Two examples of DPRs for the elementary school level are included in Appendices B.7 and B.8.)

Younger students may also need more practice and support to learn the routine of the BEP intervention. Students will not always remember to get their DPR in the morning or to check out in the afternoon. The BEP coordinator should provide the necessary support for students who are new to the intervention.

To demonstrate the differences between the BEP at the middle and the elementary school levels, we present a second example, that of Marisa Fernandez, a third-grade student. Marisa attends New Hope Elementary School. The school has had a BEP-type intervention in place for 3 years. This is the first year that Marisa has attended this school because she transferred midyear from an elementary school across town.

Marisa's school records are late in arriving, so for the first 3 weeks of her attendance, New Hope has no information about her academic or behavioral performance. However, by the fourth day of school Marisa is already demonstrating frequent, repetitive behavioral problems. She has trouble finishing tasks. She gets into arguments with her female classmates on the playground, and she frequently talks out while the teacher is presenting a lesson. Marisa's teacher, Mr. Lee, makes a request for assistance from the behavior support team.

After reviewing Mr. Lee's request for assistance, the behavior support team agrees that Marisa would be a good BEP candidate. Currently, there are only eight other students on the program, so there is plenty of room to add an additional student. In addition to reducing her behavioral problems, the BEP intervention will help Marisa become better integrated into the school. She will meet more of the New Hope staff, and she will be taught the behavioral expectations at the school. She will have positive adult contacts on a daily basis.

Before Marisa can begin the BEP, the school counselor must obtain permission from her parents. Also, as in middle school settings, baseline data should be collected. Additionally, the purpose and process of the BEP intervention must be explained to Marisa and her parents. Both of Marisa's parents are Spanish-speaking, with limited English language skills. New Hope Elementary has a high percentage of ELL (English language learner) students as well as staff who are bilingual in Spanish and English. Mr. Romero, the ELL teacher for the primary grades, is asked to attend the meeting between the school counselor, the BEP coordinator, Marisa, and her parents. Mr. Romero is able to act as an interpreter and to clear up any of Marisa's parents' concerns or questions.

Initially, her parents feel reluctant to have Marisa start the BEP. They are afraid that she is being identified as a "bad student." By working together, the school counselor and Mr. Romero are able to help them understand that the BEP will be a positive support for Marisa rather than a punishment. In the end, both parents agree to have Marisa begin the intervention. After learning that there will be opportunities to earn rewards, Marisa is excited to begin. The BEP coordinator initiates the program for Marisa on the next school day.

Prior to beginning the intervention, Mrs. Saborski, the BEP coordinator, who has been hired part-time to manage the BEP, gives Marisa a "BEP tour." That is, the afternoon before Marisa begins, Mrs. Saborski walks her through each element of the intervention. She shows Marisa where to go for check-in the next morning, and where she will pick up her DPR. She walks with Marisa to her classroom to practice giving the DPR to the teacher. By the end of the tour, Marisa feels comfortable with the new intervention.

At New Hope Elementary, the school day begins at 8:15 A.M. Students can do the BEP check-in between 7:55 and 8:15. Students are instructed to come to the library for check-in. At 7:55 A.M., Mrs. Saborski opens the doors to the library. Six of the nine BEP students check in with her between 7:55 and 8:15. The remaining three students are in kindergarten or first grade. Mrs. Saborski will go to their classrooms immediately after the 8:15 bell and check in with them individually. She found that it was difficult for the youngest children to remember to come to the library first, and that they would often be late to class when they came in for the check-in before class. The students in second through fifth grades appear to have no difficulty with checking in.

When Marisa arrives for check-in, she is shy and unsure. Mrs. Saborski asks one of the other BEP students to help Marisa. The other student reminds her where to pick up her new DPR and then stands in line with her. An example of a DPR used in Marisa's elementary school is included in Figure 3.10.

When it is Marisa's turn to check in, Mrs. Saborski praises her for remembering to come to the library. She shows Marisa where the schoolwide expectations are listed on her DPR and has Marisa read the goals to her. With Mrs. Saborski's help, Marisa writes the date at the top of her DPR. Because most elementary school students have supplies in their classrooms, check-in does not include asking students if they have materials. Like the other students, Marisa is given a "Chuckie-Buck" for checking in on time. (Chuckie, an owl, is the school's mascot.) Chuckie-Bucks are part of the schoolwide recognition and reward program at New Hope. Students can put their name on the Chuckie-Bucks and put them in the raffle box at the entrance to the

Daily Progress Report

Name: _____   2 = Good Points earned: _____

Date: _____   1 = OK   Goal: _____ Goal reached? Yes No

0 = Needs Improvement

GOALS	Reading	Math	Music	Art	Library	P.E.	Title I
Be Responsible	2 1 0	2 1 0	2 1 0	2 1 0	2 1 0	2 1 0	2 1 0
Be Kind	2 1 0	2 1 0	2 1 0	2 1 0	2 1 0	2 1 0	2 1 0
Work Hard	2 1 0	2 1 0	2 1 0	2 1 0	2 1 0	2 1 0	2 1 0
Total Points							

POSITIVE? Teacher notes: _____

POSITIVE? Parent notes: _____

Parent/guardian signature: _____

Please sign and have your child return this form on a daily basis.

FIGURE 3.10. Example of DPR used in Marisa's elementary school.

school. Every Friday, the principal draws five names from the raffle box, and each of those students receives a special prize. After Marisa has completed her check-in, she is sent to class with a prompt to be on time and to meet the schoolwide behavioral goals for the day. Often, each of the students is also sent off with a hug from Mrs. Saborski.

Once Marisa leaves, she has a few minutes before school starts. She goes directly to her third-grade classroom and is greeted by her teacher. Mr. Lee knows that Marisa is going to begin the BEP that day. He congratulates her on her good start and shows her how to put her card in the box for DPR cards on his desk. Mr. Lee waits for natural breaks in the flow of classroom activity to go over Marisa's DPR with her after each classroom transition. For example, after the students have completed morning activities, they begin their reading block. Marisa begins with silent reading. At this time, Mr. Lee talks with Marisa about the points she earned during morning activities.

The rating scale for elementary school students can be different than for middle school students. In Marisa's case, the teacher circles a "2" if Marisa has met her goal and a "0" if she has not. All of the teachers at New Hope, including the specialist teachers (e.g., music, art), have participated in an inservice on the BEP, so Marisa is able to bring her card with her to each activity she attends throughout the day.

As with the middle school, teachers are encouraged to explain their ratings to the students and to give them positive praise or Chuckie-Bucks when a student meets all of his or her goals for the class period or for the school day. If a student disputes a teacher rating, the teacher has been trained not to engage the student in a discussion regarding whether or not the rating should be changed. The teacher's rating is the final rating. In addition we have found using the language "based on your behavior, you earned" versus "based on your behavior, I am going to give you" puts the ownership of the rating on the student's behavior rather than on the teacher.

At the end of the day, Mrs. Saborski comes to each BEP student's classroom to pick up the DPR card and say good-bye. The students do not meet her in the library for check-out because of concern that some students might miss their bus. Mrs. Saborski is able to check out with each student because there are a limited number of students on the intervention and because the check-out portion of the BEP is very brief. Mrs. Saborski keeps the top copy of the DPR and makes sure that Marisa puts the second copy of her card in her backpack. Marisa's parents have been instructed to look for her DPR in her backpack when she arrives home. The check-out portion of the BEP is another chance for the students to have some positive time with a caring adult.

When Marisa gets home, her parents review the DPR. Her parents are asked to sign the card and return it. They are also encouraged to write positive comments on it. Their comments can be written in Spanish, their first language. If there is any trouble with interpretation of the comments, Mr. Romero is able to assist.

After Mrs. Saborski completes check-out for the day, she enters the BEP data into the BEP database. It is important to keep up with this on at least a weekly basis as it is critical that data are used by the behavior support team to evaluate the effectiveness of the intervention. Also, either the behavior support team or the BEP coordinator should be responsible for reporting progress to staff and parents about overall effectiveness of the program. Teachers want to know that their efforts are making a difference. There are many creative ways to make this work at an elementary school. It is up to the principal and the behavioral support team to identify the strategy that works best for their school.

WEEKLY OR TWICE-MONTHLY FEATURES

On a weekly or twice-monthly basis, there are six primary goals to meet: (1) summarize data for each BEP student; (2) prioritize students; (3) examine data to determine if a student's BEP should be continued, modified, or ended; (4) award additional "reinforcers" to deserving students; (5) discuss new potential candidates for the BEP; and (6) assign tasks to relevant staff members. Each of these goals is discussed in detail below.

Summarize Data

The power of the BEP resides in two critical elements of the intervention: first, providing continual, specific feedback and positive behavioral support to a student throughout the day, and, second, using data to make decisions. Once the data have been collected on a daily basis, it is critical to use these data for more than just a written record. It is easiest to utilize the data if one or two persons are responsible for entering the BEP data into a database on a regular basis. That is, at the end of each day, or at least at the end of each week, the BEP coordinator, or a behavior support team member, enters the percentage of points earned by each student into a BEP database (more information on databases that can be used is provided in Chapter 7). For students who have smiley faces on their DPRs, numbers should be assigned to each face. For example, a student would receive a "2" for a smiley face, a "1" for a neutral face, and a "0" for a sad face.

Once each student's data have been entered, it should be easy to create individual graphs to illustrate how well the student is doing on the BEP intervention. These graphs should be printed and brought to the behavior support team meeting, where the team can then review them.

Prioritize Students

Typically, reviewing BEP data is only one part (approximately 20 minutes) of the behavior support team meeting. In middle schools of 500 or more students, there may be as many as 30 students on the BEP intervention at one time. In-depth review of the data for each student within that limited time span will be impossible. A cursory review of all students is possible, but unlikely to produce useful results. Thus, the team should plan which students to discuss at the BEP meeting. We suggest prioritizing the students prior to beginning each behavior support team meeting.

After printing individual graphs for BEP students, the BEP coordinator can briefly review each graph. A visual inspection of each graph will quickly make evident those students who are consistently meeting their behavioral goals, those students who are consistently failing to meet their goals or to turn in their DPRs, and those students who are demonstrating variable performance. The BEP coordinator should choose two to four students of concern to prioritize for the BEP meetings. Students who are not meeting their behavioral goals or who have recently demonstrated an abrupt, negative change in their BEP performance are good prioritization candidates. Each of the "priority students" is discussed in detail at the team meeting in order to make data-based decisions regarding his or her status on the BEP and his or her behavioral support needs.

Make Data-Based Decisions

During the behavior team meeting, decisions are made whether to continue the BEP as planned, determine if modifications are necessary, or fade a student off the BEP. These decisions are based on the graphed data of each student's percentage of points (see sample graph presented in Figure 3.9). In general, if a student is consistently meeting and exceeding his or her daily point goals, no modifications are necessary. Over time, a plan for fading the student off the intervention can occur. However, if a student continually misses his or her daily point goal (e.g., meeting the goal only once or twice a week), the behavior support team will need to look at modifying the intervention or, potentially, modifying the daily point goal for a short period of time until the student can be successful on the intervention. Detailed information about how to make data-based decisions with BEP data can be found in Chapter 7.

Award Reinforcers

Sometimes the behavior support team will decide to reward a student for improvement or for consistently meeting his or her behavioral goals. Detailed information on designing reinforcements systems for the BEP is provided in Chapter 6. A simple way to provide reinforcers to students who have done well on the BEP is to provide a $1.00 coupon to the school store or snack bar.

The power of this simple reinforcement system can be increased in two ways. The coupon can be signed and hand-delivered by the principal, who praises and encourages the student for his or her behavior. A copy of the student's BEP graph can be attached to the coupon. Providing the student with a graph of his or her behavior achieves several purposes:

1. It helps the student visualize and understand his or her own behavior.
2. It helps the student understand how his or her behavior is viewed by others.
3. It helps the student realize that someone is paying close attention to his or her behavior and that there is real meaning behind the DPR that he or she turns in each day.
4. It helps the student set goals and recognize whether he or she has achieved them, or if he or she needs to continue to work harder to achieve them.

Discuss New Candidates for the BEP

Another weekly or twice-monthly responsibility of the behavior support team is to discuss new referrals to the BEP intervention. In a school in which the BEP has been fully implemented, the teaching staff will be well aware of the BEP as a resource for managing problem behavior. The staff will need to have a way to access the team. This can usually be accomplished with a simple referral form. Once a student has been referred to the BEP, the team needs to decide whether or not that student should be added to the program. The criteria mentioned earlier in this chapter can serve as a guideline for determining which students are appropriate candidates.

Additionally, the team should consider how many students are already on the BEP. When schools develop the BEP to fit their school culture, the team involved in that development should determine the maximum number of students that they can adequately manage on the BEP at one time. Once they have determined a reasonable number of students who can be served by the BEP, the behavior support team should remain true to that decision. Some schools try to respond to every behavioral concern by placing the student on the BEP. As a result, the behavior support team and the BEP coordinator get overloaded and overwhelmed, and the BEP is not as effective as it can be when it is not run beyond capacity. It is critical that the team stay within the limits established when the intervention was developed. This limit can change over time with changes in resources and/or number of people who are able to serve as the BEP coordinator.

If the BEP intervention is already filled to capacity but the behavior support team believes that a new student referral will benefit greatly from it, the team should consider whether other students are ready to be removed from the BEP. (A detailed description of strategies for fading students from the BEP is provided in Chapter 7.) A frequent mistake is to keep students on the BEP indefinitely. One goal of the BEP is to help the student learn to gain control over his or her behavior, that is, to become a good self-manager. Maintaining the student on the BEP indefinitely promotes dependence rather than independence and self-management skills.

Assign Tasks

While evaluating BEP data, the behavior support team typically generates a list of "things to do." For example, if the team decides to add a student to the BEP, one of the team members will need to set up a meeting with the parents and the student. Before the team meeting ends, a team member should be assigned to this task with a deadline of 2–4 days to complete each task. If additional supports are decided on, someone needs to be in charge of implementing those supports. If the student is to receive a reinforcement coupon, someone needs to deliver the coupon to the student.

QUARTERLY FEATURES

The critical features of the quarterly BEP process are providing feedback to the teachers and staff, and providing feedback to the students and their families. It is important to provide feedback to these two stakeholder groups for the following reasons: (1) to acknowledge the right of parents, staff, and students to be informed about their school or their child; (2) to maintain interest and involvement; (3) to recognize and encourage accomplishments; and (4) to point out needed areas of improvement (new goals) and achieve collaboration in meeting those goals.

Feedback to Teachers and Staff

Teachers and staff need to know how well the BEP intervention is running. Some questions that can be answered include: *How many students have been served on it? Is there consistent participation from students? Is there consistent participation from teachers and staff? What has been the impact on individual student behavior? What has been the impact on overall school climate? What has been working well? What is still presenting obstacles? How can the teachers and staff contribute to improving the BEP intervention? Which students deserve recognition? Which teachers and staff members deserve recognition and appreciation?*

The behavior support team can be creative about how to provide this feedback to the staff and families. One school created a bulletin called "The BEP Gazette" that was distributed to staff on a quarterly basis. The bulletin listed the students on the BEP (identified by first name only) with a brief indication of their progress, provided reminders about meetings, and gave helpful hints on basic behavior management.

The bulletin can be distributed to teachers, staff, and BEP families. It is important to preserve confidentiality, so individual students should not be mentioned by full name unless they and their parents have given their express written consent. This is true even if the student is to be recognized for improvement. Remember, while it is exciting to be recognized for one's accomplishments, not all students may want to be publicly associated with a Tier II behavior intervention.

Another way to provide feedback to teachers and staff is at staff meetings. The BEP coordinator or other representative of the behavior support team can give a report on the BEP intervention and its impact. Students and families can be provided with individual feedback at parent–teacher conferences. Both methods of providing feedback are convenient because both sets of meetings are already incorporated into the school's operating system. The behavior support team takes advantage of existing meetings to achieve this important purpose.

Some schools prefer to update students and families on a monthly basis by giving students a copy of their graph and sending a copy of the graph home to parents. This is a low-cost method to keep both parents and students involved in the intervention.

TROUBLESHOOTING PROBLEMS
WITH IMPLEMENTATION OF THE BEP

Thus far, we have provided information on how the BEP works when it runs smoothly. Students check in on a regular basis, take the DPR to their teachers throughout the day, and check out in the afternoon. The student remembers to get his or her DPR signed by a parent. This trouble-free scenario is not the case for all students. An important aspect of effectively implementing the BEP intervention involves modifying the intervention when it is not working for specific students or when the student is not participating in the program. Adaptations and elaborations to the BEP are discussed in Chapter 8.

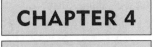

CHAPTER 4

Getting a BEP Intervention Started

Before implementing the BEP intervention, schools will want to be careful and well organized. It is critical to lay a strong foundation on which to build a sustainable intervention rather than to rush haphazardly into implementation. School administrators and the behavior support team should confirm that all the critical prerequisites are in place to produce an effective intervention that will be maintained over time. Getting carried away with the desire to "implement change now" when the necessary groundwork has not been laid will likely result in an unsatisfactory outcome, that is, no one knows what to do, how to do it, why they are doing it, or what to expect from it. Once an intervention has been tried and has failed, it can be very challenging to convince teachers and staff to give it a second chance. It is critical to demonstrate effectiveness and efficiency from the beginning of the BEP implementation.

"IS MY SCHOOL READY TO IMPLEMENT THE BEP?"

Begin by assessing whether the school, as a whole, is committed to contributing to the successful implementation of the BEP. The BEP Implementation Readiness Questionnaire (see Figure 4.1 and Appendix C.1) lists the critical features that must be in place for successful implementation of the BEP. The team of individuals who will be leading the BEP implementation should complete this questionnaire together. An administrator must be included on the team to ensure administrative support for the BEP implementation.

The team should be able to answer "Yes" to each question *prior* to BEP implementation. In addition, the team should be able to provide evidence that supports their responses. For example, if the team answers "Yes" to question 2 regarding staff commitment, then the team should be able to supply concrete evidence of staff commitment. *Was the BEP system discussed at a staff meeting? Were the staff polled regarding their interest and willingness to support the BEP? Did 80% or more of the staff agree to support the system? Can staff members accurately articulate their personal responsibilities in BEP implementation?*

In our experience, schools that have implemented a schoolwide approach to positive behavior support (PBS) are in a better position to successfully implement the BEP intervention than

Is your school ready to implement the BEP? Prior to implementation of the BEP, it is recommended that the following features be in place. Please circle the answer that best describes your school at this time.

(Yes) No   1. Our school has a schoolwide positive behavior support system in place. In essence, we have decided on three to five rules and have explicitly taught the rules to all students. We provide rewards to students for following the rules and provide mild consequences for rule infractions.

(Yes) No   2. We have secured staff commitment for implementation of the BEP. The majority of staff agree that this intervention is needed to support students at risk for serious problem behavior, and they are willing to actively participate in the intervention.

(Yes) No   3. There is administrative support for implementation of the BEP intervention. The administrative staff are committed to implementing and maintaining the BEP in our school. Administrators have allocated the necessary financial and staff resources to support implementation of the program.

(Yes) No   4. There have been no major recent changes in the school system that could hinder successful implementation of the BEP intervention. Major changes include things such as teacher strikes, high teacher or administrative turnover, or major changes in funding.

(Yes) No   5. We have made implementation of the BEP one of the school's top three priorities for this school year.

FIGURE 4.1. Example of a completed BEP Implementation Readiness Questionnaire.

schools without such Tier I prevention for behavior support. Without a schoolwide PBS system, too much time is spent on managing individual student behavior problems and the Tier II intervention is overwhelmed and ineffective.

In addition to staff agreement, administrative commitment is crucial. Administrators must be willing to participate in the development and operation of the BEP intervention. They should be willing and able to allocate the necessary personnel and financial resources to adequately support implementation. Administrators should monitor the effectiveness of the program and encourage the behavior support team to make improvements to the intervention as necessary.

Our experience in schools has taught us that implementing new interventions or attempting to change school systems will likely result in failure if the school itself is in the midst of significant change (e.g., teachers are threatening to strike, high turnover of administrative or teaching staff). When implemented consistently, the BEP is a powerful system to support students who are at risk for more serious forms of problem behavior (e.g., Fairbanks et al., 2007; Hawken, 2006; Hawken & Horner, 2003; March & Horner, 2002). If the intervention is implemented incorrectly or attempts are made to change a system that is unstable, implementation of the BEP is more likely to be unsuccessful.

Commitment to too many projects at the same time is another threat to the successful implementation of the BEP intervention. For example, a school may choose to implement the BEP, adopt a new reading curriculum, and initiate an on-site mental health clinic in the same year. With so many large projects beginning at once, the energy and effort necessary to build and sustain an effective BEP intervention may become too diluted to be effective. Thus, we recommend that implementation of the BEP be one of the school's top three priorities and that it only occur when the school is not initiating multiple new, major projects in the same year.

"HOW DO WE BUILD
SCHOOLWIDE COMMITMENT TO THE BEP INTERVENTION?"

Establishing schoolwide commitment to the BEP intervention is critical to ensuring its success. The BEP is implemented across all school settings, so the majority (at least 80%) of school staff must agree to participate in the intervention. If you are a school psychologist, counselor, behavior specialist, or other person who is trying to facilitate BEP implementation, begin by meeting with the principal and other administrators to introduce the BEP and determine their level of interest.

Once administrator support has been secured, information about the BEP should be brought to the school-based team responsible for responding to students with academic and behavioral difficulties. If there is commitment at the team level, this team should present the BEP to the whole faculty during a regularly scheduled faculty meeting. During this faculty meeting, it is essential that the administrator or a team member provide a convincing explanation for why the BEP is needed by this school at this time. We recommend that the administrator share office discipline referral data with the staff as one means to demonstrate the need for a Tier II intervention. Additionally, staff surveys may indicate that a majority of staff identified Tier II interventions as a critical need in the school, and this data could also be shared.

When attempting to build schoolwide commitment to the BEP program, we have found it very helpful to show the DVD *The Behavior Education Program: A Check-In, Check-Out Intervention for Students at Risk* (Hawken et al., 2005, available at *www.guilford.com*). This DVD visually demonstrates the critical components of the BEP intervention in a 25-minute video.

After the team has shown the BEP DVD, or has thoroughly explained the BEP intervention in a different manner, the team should provide a detailed account of the responsibilities of each teacher who participates in the BEP intervention. Once staff have received information about the BEP and the expectations for their involvement, we recommend that the whole staff vote on whether or not they are willing to participate in the intervention. (See Appendix C.2 for a voting form.)

After the staff have voted, a team member should tally the votes and determine if at least 80% of the staff have agreed to participate. If not, the administrator and other team members must engage in additional consensus building. If only a small percentage of the staff are willing to support the BEP, the intervention will fail. The staff must agree that there is a need for the BEP at their school, and they must be willing to actively participate.

THE BEP DEVELOPMENT AND IMPLEMENTATION GUIDE

After establishing that the school is ready to implement the BEP intervention, the behavior support team should meet, for at least one school day (typically during a professional development day), to create the BEP for the school. The BEP Development and Implementation Guide (see Appendix C.3) provides the structure for developing and individualizing the BEP to fit within the culture of the school. The team should work together to develop procedures and systems in answer to each question on the guide. Procedures and systems should be in place prior to beginning the BEP intervention with any one student.

Personnel Considerations

Adequate personnel time should be assigned to implement, manage, and maintain the intervention. Some schools choose to hire an educational assistant (i.e., paraprofessional) part time to lead the BEP, or assign the BEP to an educational assistant as part of his or her overall responsibilities. Responsibility for the BEP intervention must be part of a person's job description, not an added responsibility without time allocated to do the job effectively. The BEP coordinator must have no other work commitments in the half hour before school begins and after school ends. The BEP coordinator should be highly regarded by the students and interact positively and warmly with them. It is important to designate a supervisor for the BEP coordinator such as a counselor or school psychologist with experience in behavior intervention. The BEP coordinator typically requires ongoing training to work with students on the BEP. The supervisor should provide this training. More information about training needs is provided in Chapter 5.

The behavior support team should identify one or two substitutes to conduct check-in and check-out if the BEP coordinator is unavailable on a given day. It is very disappointing for students to come to school expecting to see the BEP coordinator and find that he or she is out sick for the day. Substitutes for the BEP coordinator may be the coordinator's supervisor, a special education teacher, a vice principal, or another educational assistant. This person should also have flexibility in his or her work schedule before and after school.

Location

The behavior support team should identify a location for check-in and check-out. Check-in and check-out should occur in a central, easily accessible location. At the same time, the setting should be semiprivate. Middle and high school students often prefer to avoid drawing attention to their involvement in an intervention. Conversely, elementary-age students become excited about the intervention when they realize that students on the BEP receive extra attention from the BEP coordinator. The location of check-in/check-out must fit with the logistics of your school. It can be located in the counselor's office, library, vice principal's office, or any other room that works well for the school.

Developing a user-friendly Daily Progress Report (DPR) is important for successful implementation of the BEP. The DPR is a tool for teachers to provide quick feedback on the student's behavior throughout the day. DPRs should not require teachers to write long narratives about the student's behavior but rather provide simple, numerical ratings of behavior. We strongly recommend that schools include their schoolwide expectations on the DPR to provide additional practice and feedback for these students who need it most. More detailed information on designing DPRs is provided in Chapter 6.

Reinforcement System

A critical component of the BEP intervention is to regularly provide reinforcement for appropriate behavior. Reinforcement for students who display chronic behavior problems is controversial for some school personnel. Many staff members have asked, "Why should students who are engaging in problem behavior be targeted to receive extra acknowledgment and reinforcement?" Since students who qualify for BEP support have not made progress with the schoolwide Tier I prevention efforts, universally implemented strategies are not effective or adequate for these students. Therefore, these students need additional reinforcement and feedback to get their behavior on the right track. Experience tells us that if we do not intervene early with problem behavior, the behavior will worsen over time.

In developing a reinforcement system for the BEP, it is important to emphasize the social aspects of the intervention. This includes increasing adult attention and can also involve utilizing reinforcers that increase positive peer attention. In order to reduce the expense of reinforcers, we recommend using reinforcers that do not incur a financial cost (e.g., spending time with a preferred adult or friend, or engaging in an easily accessible activity, such as additional computer or gym time). More information about developing an effective reinforcement system is provided in Chapter 6.

Referral System

In Chapter 3, we described the students who are appropriate for the BEP. The behavior support team should develop a school-specific referral system prior to BEP implementation. The team should identify decision criteria for assigning students to the BEP. A parental permission form should be created. Finally, the team should identify decision criteria to determine if students who received BEP support during the previous school year should be placed on the BEP at the beginning of the following school year. Most schools prefer to allow students time to become acquainted with their new teachers and classroom(s) before beginning the BEP. At times, a change in classroom or teacher results in a significant difference in the student's behavior, and he or she no longer needs the support of the BEP. The goal is not to wait for the student to fail (i.e., not provide BEP support until he or she engages in problem behavior), but rather to first allow the new teacher an opportunity to get to know the student and offer behavior support within the classroom.

System to Manage Data and Fade Intervention

During the professional development day, the behavior support team must also decide how to summarize and graph the daily data. In Chapter 7, we describe computer program options for summarizing data. Once the data are evaluated on a regular basis, the team will need to decide when it is appropriate to fade students off the intervention. Sometimes, the end of the school year serves as a natural fade period for the students, and they do not receive BEP support the following school year. Additionally, given that only a limited number of students can be supported on the BEP at one time, it is important to systematically fade students off the intervention once they have been successful and demonstrated that they no longer need the support. Detailed information on fading students off the BEP intervention is provided in Chapter 7.

System to Address Training Needs

The final questions from the BEP Development and Implementation Guide are related to staff, student, and parent training needs. Each person who participates or contributes to the intervention must deeply understand and agree to his or her responsibilities. A comprehensive plan for addressing training needs is presented in Chapter 5.

A completed sample version of the BEP Development and Implementation Guide is presented in Figure 4.2.

1. Determine personnel needs and logistics.
   - Who will be the BEP coordinator?

   Ms. Gomez—ELL paraprofessional

   - Who will supervise the BEP coordinator?

   Mrs. Carroll—school psychologist

   - Who will check students in and out when coordinator is absent? (Name **at least two** people who can substitute for the coordinator.)

   Mr. Singh—special ed. teacher, Mrs. Hannon—counselor

   - Where will check-in and check-out occur?

   Small room outside Mrs. Carroll's office

   - What is the maximum number of students that can be served on the BEP at one time?

   We will start with three to five, see how it goes, problem-solve issues/concerns, then slowly add up to 20 students.

   - What is the name of the BEP at your school and what will the Daily Progress Report be called?

   ROAR = Reinforcement of Appropriate Responses
   DPR = Wild Card

2. Develop a Daily Progress Report (DPR).
   - What will the behavioral expectations be?

   Keep your hands, feet, and other objects to self (KYHFOOTY), be on task, follow directions first time + added work completion to schoolwide rules
       There will be two DPRs—upper grade and lower grade

   - Are the expectations positively stated?

   Yes

   - Is the DPR teacher-friendly? How often are teachers asked to rate the student's behavior?

   Yes, lower grade = 4 rating periods, upper grade = 7 grading periods

   - Is the DPR age-appropriate and does it include a range of scores?

   Yes, 0, 1, 2 scale

   - Are the data easy to summarize?

   Yes

3. Develop a reinforcement system for students on the BEP.
   - What will the students daily point goal be?

   Bare minimum score = 70%; students who receive higher scores will receive more points on their credit card

(cont.)

FIGURE 4.2. Example of a completed BEP Development and Implementation Guide.

- What reinforcers will students receive for checking in (e.g., praise and lottery ticket)?
Praise and lottery ticket for end-of-week drawing. Public posting of drawing winner and small mystery motivator prize for student who won the drawing. Student can draw either a banana or coconut off a tree for the mystery motivator prize.

- What reinforcers will students receive for checking out **AND** meeting their daily point goal?
Praise, daily spinner for meeting goal and for longer term rewards— $\geq 70\%$ = 1 point on credit card, $\geq 80\%$ = 2 points on credit card, $\geq 90\%$ = 3 points on credit card, 100 % = 4 points to be spent at school store

- How will you ensure students do not become bored with the reinforcers?
School store items to be changed frequently and change items on the spinner

- What are the consequences for students who receive major and minor referrals?
Students cannot exchange points for items if they receive a referral nor receive daily spinner.

4. Develop a referral system.
   - How will students be referred to the BEP? What are the criteria for placing students on the BEP?
   Referred by teacher or after receiving three minor behavior referrals. Data from behavior logs (in-class consequences) will be examined to also determine eligibility.

   - What does the parental consent form look like for students participating in the BEP?
   Will revise example provided in the training

   - What is the process for screening students who transfer into the school?
   Behavior support team will review behavior data from other school. Will determine if BEP is needed. In most cases student will start without BEP support to acclimate to the school.

   - What is the process for determining whether students will begin the next school year on the BEP?
   Most students will start the new year without BEP support to get used to new teachers/classrooms. In a few cases teacher may advocate that it's necessary for student to be successful and student will be placed on BEP after first week of school.

5. Develop a system for managing the daily data.
   - Which computer program will be used to summarize data?
   Check-In, Check-Out SWIS data system [see Chapter 7]

   - Which team in the school will examine the daily BEP data and how frequently will it be examined? (note: data should be examined at least twice-monthly.)
   Multidisciplinary team will carve out 20–30 minutes every other week for BEP data evaluation.

   - Who is responsible for summarizing the data and bringing it to team meetings?
   Ms. Gomez will summarize data and attend BEP portion of the behavior support team meetings.

   - How frequently will data be shared with the whole staff?
   Once per quarter

   - How frequently will data be shared with parents?
   A graph will be sent home to parents monthly. Parents will also receive a longer term graph during parent–teacher conferences.

(cont.)

FIGURE 4.2. *(cont.)*

6. Plan to fade students off the intervention.
   - What are the criteria for fading students off the BEP?
   Tentatively, we will evaluate all students every quarter. On average, if student receives 80% or more across 6 weeks, fading will be considered. Teachers will be consulted prior to fading.

   - How will the BEP be faded and who will be in charge of helping students fade off the BEP?
   Students will self-monitor their progress and reduce the number of check-ins and check-outs. Over time, students will check in at the beginning of the week and check out at the end of the week. Ms. Gomez will be in charge of teaching students how to self-monitor and other aspects of fading.

   - How will graduation from the BEP be celebrated?
   Lunch time party with small cake, parents, teacher(s), and support staff. Students will receive diploma signed by behavior support team.

   - What incentives and supports will be put in place for students who graduate from the program?
   Quarterly "alumni" parties for students who graduate and do not receive ODRs

7. Plan for staff training.
   - Who will train staff on the BEP?
   Behavior support team using protocol outlined in BEP book

   - Who will provide teachers with individual coaching if the BEP is not being implemented as planned?
   Mrs. Catrell—principal

   - Who will provide yearly booster sessions about the purpose and key features in implementing the BEP?
   Behavior support team

8. Plan for student and parent training.
   - Who will meet with students to train them on the intervention?
   Ms. Gomez will meet with student following baseline collection to train them. Role playing will be used along with giving the student a tour of how/where to check in, check out and how to get teacher feedback.

   - How will parents be trained on the intervention?
   Mrs. Carroll, school psychologist, will either meet with parents or provide information over the phone about how to participate. She will also be in charge of getting parental permission. As Ms. Gomez becomes more comfortable with implementing the BEP, she may also be involved in training parents.

FIGURE 4.2. *(cont.)*

BUDGET

The budget for initial and sustained implementation of the BEP will vary depending on the size of the school, number of students involved, and amount of employee hours needed for check-in/check-out, data entry, team meeting coordination, and other BEP coordinator tasks. Our goal is not to stipulate a specific dollar amount needed to implement the BEP, but to suggest the budget categories and offer at least one operating model budget. The key message is that adequate resources must be allocated to support and maintain successful implementation of the BEP.

Budget categories and estimated annual costs per category from one middle school with approximately 500 students are provided in Figure 4.3.

Budget category	Category description	Example amount
Personnel		
	BEP coordinator (9–13 hours per week)	Per district pay scale
Materials		
	BEP forms on NCR paper	$250
	School supplies	$200*
Incentives		
	Small rewards	$500*

FIGURE 4.3. Sample BEP budget. *These items can also be donated from local department stores, grocery stores, and businesses.

FINAL CONSIDERATIONS PRIOR TO BEP IMPLEMENTATION

A crucial component of an effective system of behavior support is that the key stakeholders are aware of it and are willing to use it. If teachers do not know that this source of support exists, they will not make referrals, and consequently very few students will be placed on the BEP. In addition, if teachers and staff have not been adequately trained on the BEP, they will not know how to respond when a student brings a DPR for their feedback. It only takes a few inconsistent or negative responses from an adult for a student to lose interest in cooperating with the BEP. Lack of communication among the teachers and staff in the building could put an end to the BEP intervention before it has a fair chance to work. This is why obtaining teacher and staff commitment prior to BEP implementation is essential.

Equally important, students must understand what the BEP intervention is and how it works. This is true not only for the students on the BEP, but for all the students in the school. When all the students in the school know about the BEP, they can support their friends who are on the BEP. The intervention becomes part of the school culture. When only a few students know about it, the program may be viewed with skepticism or ridicule. It may be viewed as one of those things they do for the "bad kids." Students tend to avoid interventions that set them apart or give them a label.

The BEP must become a positive part of the school culture. How can this be accomplished?

1. *Begin by giving the BEP a high profile within the school.* Explain the BEP intervention to teachers and staff at the first staff development meeting of the year. Continue to provide this same inservice in subsequent years. Returning teachers and staff will benefit from the reminder. New teachers will be immediately incorporated into the system. Also, explain the BEP intervention to the student body at the beginning of each school year.

2. *Always stress the positive aspects of the BEP intervention.* Talk about the BEP frequently in staff meetings. Give the teachers and staff quarterly updates on BEP student progress. Talk about the BEP at student pep assemblies.

3. *Ensure that the BEP is viewed as a positive support, not a punishment.* Publicly recognize students for their accomplishments on the BEP (with their permission). Use the BEP as a way for students to earn privileges. Publicly recognize teachers who contribute to the BEP. Publicly recognize and thank behavior support team members for their hard work on the BEP.

4. *Provide regular feedback.* It is important to provide regular feedback to the students, staff, and families. We all are more likely to believe in an intervention when we can see the real impact of the program. Regular specific feedback to each group of key stakeholders in the BEP process is essential.

CHAPTER 5

Roles, Responsibilities, and Training Needs Related to Implementing the BEP

DEANNE A. CRONE, LEANNE S. HAWKEN, and K. SANDRA MACLEOD

Prior to implementing the BEP intervention, schools must understand the roles and responsibilities of everyone involved in the intervention and delineate how BEP training will be conducted. This includes the BEP coordinator, behavior support team members, administrators, teaching staff, parents, and students. To a great extent, the success of the BEP intervention hinges on the effectiveness of the BEP coordinator. Therefore, the BEP coordinator must receive adequate training on implementing and managing the intervention. Staff members should receive training on the features of the BEP intervention and on how to implement it within their classroom or school setting. Students and parents should receive training on their responsibilities and on how to successfully participate in the intervention. Finally, the behavior support team will require training on how to use data for decision making.

The purpose of this chapter is to describe the distinct roles and responsibilities of each person or group of persons involved in the BEP intervention, as well as to delineate the critical elements to be included during the corresponding training sessions.

BEP COORDINATOR

Roles and Responsibilities

The primary responsibilities of the BEP coordinator are to (1) lead morning check-in; (2) lead afternoon check-out; (3) enter DPR data into a graphing program at least once per week; (4) maintain records in centrally located, confidential location; (5) create BEP graphs for team

K. Sandra MacLeod, PhD, is a recent graduate of the Special Education Department, University of Utah, Salt Lake City, Utah.

TABLE 5.1. BEP Coordinator's Time Allocation

Task	Frequency	Duration	Total time/week
Lead morning check-in	5 times per week	30–45 minutes	150–225 minutes
Lead afternoon check-out	5 times per week	20–30 minutes	100–150 minutes
Enter BEP data onto spreadsheet	1 time per week	30 minutes	30 minutes
Maintain records	5 times per week	15 minutes	75 minutes
Prioritize BEP students	1 time per week	20 minutes	20 minutes
Process BEP referrals	As needed	10–20 minutes	10–20 minutes
Create BEP graphs for team meetings	1 time per week	30 minutes	30 minutes
Gather supplemental information	As needed	30–90 minutes	30–90 minutes
Attend behavior support team meetings	1 time per week	30–45 minutes	30–45 minutes
Complete tasks from BEP meetings	As needed	60–120 minutes	60–120 minutes
		TOTAL TIME	9–13 hours

meetings; (6) prioritize students for team meetings; (7) gather supplemental information for meetings; (8) attend team meetings; and (9) complete any tasks assigned at the meetings.

An educational assistant can carry out the responsibilities of the BEP coordinator. Most schools employ one or several full-time educational assistants. The job responsibilities of an educational assistant tend to be more flexible than those of a teacher or administrator. Coordinating the BEP intervention should take about 9–13 hours each week, depending on the size of the school and the number of students supported on the intervention. The tasks of the BEP coordinator and the necessary time allotted are illustrated in Table 5.1. A weekly behavior support team meeting is assumed. If the team meets less frequently, time allocation should be adjusted accordingly.

Leading Morning Check-In and Afternoon Check-Out

Morning check-in is the BEP students' first point of contact with the school for the day. On a daily basis, morning check-in provides the students with an ideal opportunity to start the day well. Afternoon check-out is the BEP students' last point of contact with the school. It is an opportunity to send students home with a positive attitude and a reason to look forward to the next school day. *The person who does check-in and check-out must be someone whom the students respect, enjoy, and trust.* This person should be enthusiastic, positive, and friendly. When students look forward to seeing a person, they are much more likely to cooperate by checking in and checking out on a regular basis than if they find the BEP coordinator to be dismissive, harsh, or punishing. Another important characteristic of the BEP coordinator is that he or she must be able to multitask and manage moderate-sized groups of students. We have seen BEP coordinators who become frazzled when working with more than five students or who struggle because they do not enjoy the quick pace of the check-in and check-out process.

The logistics of leading check-in and check-out may seem complicated or overwhelming at first. All that is needed, however, is to establish a simple, accessible, predictable routine. Once the BEP coordinator has established the routine and each BEP student has been taught the routine, daily check-in and check-out will become almost automatic.

Morning check-in should not last more than 30 minutes and should end before the first bell rings for school to begin. Students should not use participation in the BEP as an excuse for being late to their first class! We have found that some of the younger elementary school students need to have their DPRs delivered directly to their classroom as it is difficult for them to remember to check in in the morning. Also, after the morning check-in time, the BEP coordinator must determine if students who have not checked in are indeed absent or have simply forgotten to check in. If the student forgot to check in, the BEP coordinator should deliver the DPR and then plan to reteach the process of checking in. Afternoon check-out should be even briefer, approximately 15–20 minutes. Many students will only have a few minutes between the dismissal bell and the time that their bus leaves the school building. The BEP coordinator should collaborate with the bus monitors to ensure that no students are left behind while doing BEP check-out.

Morning check-in consists of the following activities:

1. Greet each student individually.
2. Collect the signed (by parents) DPR from the previous day.
3. In middle and high school settings, check to see if student has loose-leaf paper, pens, pencils, and other necessary items for the day (provide extras to the student if necessary).
4. Make sure that the student takes a new DPR, signs it, and dates it.
5. Prompt student to have a good day and meet his or her BEP goals.
6. Give student a rewards ticket (if available within the school's reinforcement system) for checking-in successfully.

The BEP coordinator should keep a BEP checklist of both the check-in and check-out process. For middle and high school settings, this checklist will include places for the BEP coordinator to mark whether the student was prepared for the day (e.g., had a pencil, paper, and daily planner), whether the DPR was brought back signed from the parent/guardian, and a place to write the percentage of points the student earned at the end of the day. In elementary school settings, we have found that most students keep supplies in their desks in their classrooms so checking for supplies is not a necessary part of check-in. (Sample check-in and check-out checklists for elementary and secondary settings are included in Appendices D.1 and D.2.)

Entering DPR Data and Maintaining Records

The DPRs, and the corresponding data, are helpful only to the extent that they are used. Completed and signed DPRs that are allowed to pile up week after week are useful only for filling up file drawer space. However, DPRs entered into a database on a daily or weekly basis can be used to monitor student progress, make data-based intervention decisions, and evaluate outcomes. A simple database can be created in Excel. Additional information regarding options for a BEP data management system is presented in Chapter 7. When data is entered on a weekly basis, it should take less than 60 minutes to complete (depending on the number of students supported on the BEP).

It is important to keep well-organized files. After the students' percentage point data have been recorded on the check-in, check-out sheet, each DPR should be filed separately into each student's file folder. Any other information relevant to the BEP (e.g., BEP graphs, consent forms from parents, or teacher interview) should be kept in individual students' files as well. The files should be orderly so that it is easy to locate information. Maintaining the files should require 15 minutes or less per day.

Information regarding a student's behavior and treatment for that behavior is confidential information. While the student's files should be accessible for the behavior support team members involved in working with the student, care should be taken to maintain the student's confidentiality. The files should be kept in a locked filing cabinet when not in use. A student's file should never be left lying out on a table or desk where other students or unrelated staff might have access to it.

Creating BEP Graphs for BEP Team Meetings

Prior to the behavior support team meeting, the coordinator should create a BEP graph for each student on the program. Printing graphs on recycled paper will save a great deal of paper over the course of the year. Putting multiple graphs on a page will further increase the amount of paper saved.

The coordinator can choose to graph only the data from the previous week or 2 weeks or to include students' data from a longer period of time. Whichever method is chosen, the data should be presented in the same manner for each student. Illustrating short-term data for some students and long-term data for other students may create confusion and errors in data interpretation by the behavior support team.

The greater part of behavior support team meetings will revolve around the "priority students." The BEP coordinator may feel that it is more efficient to only distribute graphs of the "priority students" to the team members, rather than a packet of graphs for all of the BEP students. In this case, the coordinator may find it useful to keep a master copy of all the student graphs in case questions regarding nonpriority students arise.

Prioritizing Students and Gathering Supplemental Information for BEP Team Meetings

Prior to the behavior support team meeting, the BEP coordinator should review data graphs for each of the BEP students. Many of the students will be doing well on the program, consistently meeting their goals from day to day. Other students may be performing poorly or may experience a sudden decline in performance. Some of the same students may be receiving detention or suspensions, or have poor attendance. The BEP coordinator will have access to this information as well. It is important to understand what is happening with these students and to determine if the students need additional supports.

The BEP coordinator should prioritize two to four students for discussion at each behavior support team meeting. In addition to providing BEP graphs for each priority student, the coordinator can generate a copy of the student's detention/ODR record, attendance record, or progress reports. This supplemental information can aid the behavior support team in making data-based intervention decisions. The BEP coordinator may also choose to prioritize a student in order to follow up on a previous decision or discussion.

The BEP coordinator can gather information from teachers when the intervention is not working for a particular student. This could involve asking teachers why the student is consistently not meeting goals or problem solving with the teacher about why the student is not attending check-out. Members of the behavior support team may also be involved in gathering this information.

Attending Behavior Support Team Meetings

The BEP coordinator should attend the behavior support team meetings whenever BEP data are discussed. Reviewing BEP data is typically only one part of a behavior support team meeting, and therefore the BEP coordinator does not need to attend the entire meeting. In some schools, BEP data are discussed every other week during the first 20 minutes of the behavior support team meeting. The BEP coordinator attends that portion of the meeting and brings graphs for the team to review. The BEP coordinator brings the critical information to the meeting so that the team can discuss each student and decide on a plan of action. The entire team then shares in the tasks or responsibilities generated at the team meetings.

Completing Any Tasks Assigned at the Behavior Support Team Meetings

Multiple tasks may be generated from the team meeting. If a new student is added to the BEP, one of the team members will need to contact the parents for permission to participate and to set up an orientation meeting. If a priority student is not succeeding on the BEP, the team may decide to provide additional behavioral support to him or her. For example, the team may propose a schedule change, curriculum assessment, or instruction on a behavioral skill. Once a plan of action has been decided on, someone needs to implement the plan. The team members will share responsibility for coordinating the implementation of additional behavioral supports. Some of the responsibility for these tasks will fall to the BEP coordinator.

Training

BEP coordinators are typically paraprofessionals (e.g., educational assistants), supervised by a school psychologist or school counselor. Training for the BEP coordinator is delivered by the specialist or administrator who is leading the BEP effort at the school and who deeply understands the BEP intervention and process. Typically, this trainer is a school psychologist, counselor, special education teacher, or vice principal. The BEP coordinator should receive an initial training session on how to coordinate and manage the multiple components of the intervention. Ongoing training should occur as necessary. Figure 5.1 delineates the content that should be addressed during BEP coordinator training.

- Overall PBS structure of the school
  - Schoolwide rules, how and when taught
  - Other Tier II interventions
- Importance of student and BEP coordinator relationship
  - Positive relationship cornerstone to the effectiveness of the BEP
  - Goal = 5:1 positive to negative ratio of interactions
- Confidentiality and roles of coordinator versus counselor/school psychologist
  - Where should student files be kept? Ensuring all staff do not have access to files, etc.
  - Which staff members should know which students are on the BEP?
  - BEP coordinator is not a counselor—importance of being supportive and referring to teacher, principal, or school psychologist if problem is severe.
- Check-in procedures
  - When and where check-in occurs
  - How to greet students—varying positive things to say at check-in
  - Managing multiple students. Provide information on what to do if students do not check in.

An Example of BEP Check-In Procedures

Students check in with BEP coordinator either before school or at the beginning of school. When students check in, make sure to greet them happily. Ask them how they are doing and praise them for checking in. Ask if they have their DPR signed from the previous day. Praise them if they return it signed. Have student write his or her name, date, and goal on their new DPR and give it to them to take to class. For students who need help, write this information for them. Remind them when to check out and encourage them to do their personal best in class.

If students don't check in after 20 minutes, take their DPRs to them to see if they are absent. If they are at school, ask them why they didn't check in, give them their DPR, and encourage them to do a good job. Check in later if the student is not at school to see if he or she arrived late.

- Structure of the DPR
  - How to summarize scores
  - Required components (e.g., rating and teacher signature) versus optional components (e.g., additional positive comments)
- Check-out procedures
  - When and where check-out occurs
  - Structure of the reinforcement system
  - Procedure for sending DPRs home with students for parent signature
  - What to do if student does not check out

An Example of BEP Check-Out Procedures

Take a moment with each student to go over how his or her day went based on his or her DPR. It's important to focus on the positive, and help them feel they can succeed in the future. Then calculate their daily percentages to see if they made their goal. If they do, they spin a spinner for a small prize. For a long-term reinforcement idea, after students meet their daily goals for 10 consecutive days, they can pick a prize from a reinforcement menu. (See Chapter 6 for more reinforcement ideas.) The students then take the top copy home to get signed, and the bottom copy stays at school.

- Data entry and graph development
  - What data to enter and how to enter it
  - How often are data to be entered?
  - How often graphed?
- Attending team meetings
  - Bring graphs
  - Help prioritize students to talk about and students who need additional reinforcement

(cont.)

FIGURE 5.1. BEP coordinator training.

- Training students on the BEP
  - How to teach social skills/role-play with students
- Training parents on the BEP
  - Calling parents on the phone

Other Topics Covered during BEP Coordinator Training

- Basic principles of applied behavior analysis/behavior intervention
  - Setting Events, Antecedents, Behavior, Consequences
  - Main functions of problem behavior—why students act out
    - Escape, attention, obtaining tangible items/activities, or self-stimulatory
  - Basic principles of reinforcement
    - How to identify reinforcers for students
- Managing confrontations

BEP Coordinator Troubleshooting the BEP

Tardy to school
- Find out why student is late.
- Give a sticker for days on time and reward for a certain number of days on time (does not have to be consecutive).
- Set up self-monitoring program by having student record days on time and receive reward for a certain number of days on time (does not have to be consecutive).
- Praise the student every time he or she is on time for school.

Absences
- Check with home—find out why student is missing school.
- Is student staying home to avoid academic activity? If yes, student needs help in improving the academic skill.
- Inform parent about attendance laws.
- Help the student find an enjoyable school activity.
- Set an attendance goal with student and have a reward for a certain number of days at school (does not have to be consecutive).
- Talk to the student one-on-one about why it's important to come to school.
- Praise the student each time he or she is at school.

Student not checking in
- Students get a sticker for each check-in—earns small reward for _____ days of check-in (not consecutive).
- Check in with a buddy.
- Have a raffle ticket for check-in.
- Surprise drawing—on random days, have a special drawing for students who check in and check out.
- Put a "sticky note" on his or her desk as a reminder to check in or give him or her a note for his or her backpack.
- Praise the student for remembering to check in.

Student not checking out
- Ask the student why he or she is not checking out—make sure he or she has the time to check out, etc.
- Check out with buddy (both earn rewards).
- Give raffle tickets for check-out.
- Fun, quick, activity every now and then on a day student checks out.
- Praise the student for remembering to check out.
- Special reward for checking out—special home note.
- Surprise drawing—see above.
- Have a "sticky note" reminder to check out on his or her desk.

(cont.)

FIGURE 5.1. *(cont.)*

Complaining/pouting
- Always take note of and reinforce appropriate behavior with specific praise statements such as "Thanks for taking responsibility for that!"
- Set up a time when the student can talk to you about what he or she thinks is unfair (should be during student's free time, i.e., recess).
- Practice (i.e., role-play) accepting feedback on the DPR.
- Make sure the student knows that his or her behavior *earns* what he or she receives on the DPR.
- At check-in, precorrect for appropriate behavior when receiving feedback on the DPR.
- Problem-solve (with older students) about a situation that keeps happening.

Stealing/changing scores
- Set up a program where a student can earn extra stickers for appropriate behavior.
- Take away points for stealing (tickets, reinforcers, etc.).
- Explain that students will not earn points or make their goal when they steal or are dishonest.

Lost Daily Progress Report
- Tell students they can get a new report right away.
- If this happens often, find out if student is having consistent "bad days."
- Is the student enjoying participating in the BEP program?
- Give the student a small basket or a folder that the student and teacher can find easily.

FIGURE 5.1. *(cont.)*

Because the BEP coordinator will train students on the check-in/check-out process, he or she should be familiar with the student training scripts provided in Figure 5.2. Prior to working directly with students, the BEP coordinator can role-play the student training process with his or her supervisor. The supervisor should observe the BEP coordinator for the first two or three sessions of student training and provide constructive feedback.

The BEP coordinator should also play a role in assessing students' preferences for reinforcers. A key feature of the BEP intervention is the provision of reinforcement to students for meeting their goals. If a student consistently misses the benchmark for his daily point goal, one of the first questions asked is whether or not the reinforcement component of the intervention has been implemented as planned. As a follow-up question, the BEP coordinator can assess whether or not the student considers the reinforcers to be rewarding and desirable. If not, the reinforcers should be changed to reflect the student's interests and preferences. The BEP coordinator should understand the basic theoretical principles of reinforcement and punishment and also understand that students will become tired of the reinforcers if they are not varied or changed regularly. More information on choosing effective reinforcers is provided in Chapter 6.

We have noticed that BEP coordinators often repeat the same phrases to students during check-in and check-out. Just as students will grow weary of receiving the same reinforcers (e.g., every day they receive a sticker or a pencil for meeting their daily point goal), they will grow tired of repetitive interactions with the BEP coordinator. Figure 5.3 lists a variety of phrases to use during check-in and check-out.

We are frequently asked how the BEP coordinator manages to check in and check out 20–30 students per day. The BEP coordinator must be skilled in managing groups of students and also in managing individual students who may be engaging in problem behavior. Part of the initial training should include teaching the BEP coordinator effective routines for check in and check out. For example, it may help to limit the number of students allowed to stand at the BEP

Teaching Students How to Participate in the BEP

The purpose of this lesson plan is to teach students who are new to the BEP the expectations of the program and how to accept feedback. You'll be giving students many opportunities to see, hear, and perform the expectation correctly, and a few examples of what not to do. (Plan on about 15 minutes for this activity and have a copy of the DPR to show the student.)

First step: Introduce the student to the program and give a brief explanation of what you are going to talk about. Say something like "Today we're going to learn about the Behavior Education Program. This will help you be more successful in school and we're going to practice today so that you'll know how to be really good at doing this and you can earn all your points."

Second step: Show the student the DPR and starting at the top, go through each component of the report. Describe the meaning of each score for each expectation. You can say something like this: "This is the Daily Progress Report. Look at what is on it: it has the school expectations and some numbers. The numbers are (say numbers) and here are what the numbers mean. For the rule 'Follow Directions,' '2' means that you followed directions, etc., a '1' means you had some trouble, and a '0' means you didn't follow directions."

Ask the student to demonstrate the expectations for a rule (e.g., "Staying on task"). Use lots of praise for demonstrating the expectation and circle the 2 on the DPR example. Practice another expectation if necessary.

Third step: Show how the points are added up to give a score for the day and what the student's goal will be. Use more detail in this section for the older students. Tell them they need to pick up their DPR every day before school or after checking in with the teacher, and they will need to return them to you at the end of the day (give time).

Teaching Students How to Accept Feedback on Their DPR
Feedback at Check-Out

To practice receiving feedback about a poor DPR at check-out, you can teach students how to react to pretend examples of how to act and examples of how not to act.

Steps:
- Fill out a DPR for yourself and tell the student that you are going to pretend that this is yours.
- Give yourself 0's and some 1's so you don't make your goal. Show the student the report and talk about what it means. (Did not stay on task, follow directions, etc. I want to make my goal. . . .)
- Let the student know you are going to act in different ways when you see this report.
- Ask him or her to see if he or she can tell a difference between what we should do and what we should not do when we get a not very good DPR. He or she can show you by giving you a "thumbs-up" for the right way to act or a "thumbs-down" for the wrong way to act after each situation. ("Is this the way you should act?")

Act out these scenarios:
- Act very upset—cry, or say something like "That's stupid!" ("Thumbs-up or thumbs-down?")
- Say "I'm upset I didn't make my goal, but I'll try harder tomorrow." ("Thumbs-up or thumbs-down?")
- Act out being angry and yelling that it isn't fair, and that the teacher made a mistake, etc. ("Thumbs-up or thumbs-down?")
- Say something about how you wish you could have made your goal, but can still make your week if you try harder to follow directions, etc. ("Thumbs-up or thumbs-down?")

Role play of examples:
- You be the student and demonstrate getting an unsatisfactory DPR and handling it correctly. Ask the student to be the person giving feedback on the DPR. (Ask him or her if he or she has kept hands, feet, and other objects to him- or herself.)
- Ask the student to demonstrate correctly handling a poor DPR. (Use the "thumbs-up" and lots of praise and encouragement.)

Do not allow the student to practice nonexamples of correct behavior.

FIGURE 5.2. Student training scripts.

Things to say at check in

- Wow! You brought back your DPR signed!
- You're here on time again—great!
- Looks like you're all set to go.
- It's great to see you this morning.
- Looks like you're ready for a good day.
- You're off to a good start.
- You look so nice this morning.
- You look happy to be here this morning.
- I like the way you said "good morning."
- Thanks for coming to check in.
- Sounds like you had a good weekend.
- We missed you yesterday [if student was absent], nice to see you today.

Things to say at check-out

- You had a great [awesome, terrific, etc.] day!
- You're right on target.
- Your mom/dad is going to be so proud of you.
- You're really working hard!
- You are such a good student.
- You made your goal—wow!
- Looks like today didn't go so well—I know you can do it tomorrow.
- I know it was a tough day—thanks for coming to check out.
- We all have bad days once and awhile—I know you can do better tomorrow.
- You look a little frustrated—what happened? [If a student looks upset take a few minutes to "just listen."]

FIGURE 5.3. Tips for providing feedback during check-in, during check-out, and in class.

coordinator table at one time and expect other students to stay behind a line that is taped on the floor. For older students, the BEP coordinator may be able to check-in and check-out more than two students at a time. The BEP coordinator could sit at a kidney-shaped table while three or four students show they have their materials for the day, gather their DPRs, write their names on them, and turn in their DPRs from the previous day. Students who require more individualized attention can be supported after the check-in process is complete. The key to making check-in and check-out work for multiple students is developing and teaching effective routines to make the process manageable and predictable.

In addition to teaching check-in and check-out routines, BEP coordinators should have knowledge of basic behavior management techniques and how to diffuse confrontations between students. They should be taught when and how to seek help from other school personnel if student behavior is severe or extreme. Along with the entire school staff, BEP coordinators should have some knowledge of the functions of problem behavior. That is, they should understand the primary reasons why students act out, which include to obtain peer attention, to obtain adult attention, to escape an aversive activity, academic subject; or social situation; or to have access to a tangible object (e.g., favorite toy) they desire. If BEP coordinators understand the basic functions of problem behavior, they can better help the behavior support team modify the BEP intervention if it is ineffective for an individual student. More information about the functions of problem behavior and how the BEP can be modified to support different functions is presented in Chapter 8.

BEHAVIOR SUPPORT TEAM

Roles and Responsibilities

The primary responsibilities of the behavior support team members are to (1) attend weekly or biweekly meetings; (2) contribute to decisions regarding individual BEP students; (3) conduct orientation meetings with students and families; (4) gather supplemental information on individual students; (5) contribute to student/staff development workshops and feedback sessions on the BEP; and (6) complete any tasks assigned at the BEP meeting.

The behavior support team should incorporate a certain critical mix of individuals, including an administrator and a representative sample of the school's personnel. It is also helpful to have several individuals on the team who are knowledgeable about behavioral issues and who have had experience working with students at risk for severe problem behavior. Some schools choose to include each of their special education teachers on the behavior support team. The actual size of the team will vary from school to school. We suggest limiting the size of the team to a maximum of eight in order to facilitate the ease of decision making and planning.

The team should decide how to best use their time at each meeting. We suggest creating a standard agenda that can be used at each meeting (see Figure 5.4 for a sample agenda). At each meeting, the team should discuss the two to four "priority students," whose BEP graphs and supplemental information should be reviewed.

For each student, the behavior support team should make one of four decisions: (1) remove from BEP, (2) continue to monitor progress on BEP, (3) provide additional (minor) behavioral supports or modifications, or (4) conduct comprehensive function-based assessment and develop an intensive intervention.

After priority students have been discussed, the team will discuss any new referrals and determine if the newly referred student is an appropriate candidate for the BEP intervention. Once new referrals have been discussed, the team can turn their attention to deciding which students should receive recognition for consistently meeting their goals over the past week or for demonstrating a significant improvement on the BEP intervention. These students can be rewarded by having the principal share the graph with the student and congratulate him or her on consistently meeting goals. Some schools combine this recognition with a $1.00 coupon to the school store or a similar reward. Finally, if any time remains, the BEP team members can discuss any other issues relevant to the BEP intervention or other BEP students.

Finally, BEP team members must understand how to modify the BEP if it is not working. Chapter 8 provides information on how to modify the BEP when it is not working. This informa-

---

Date: _____   Note taker: _____

Team members present: _____

List of priority students:

#1   Discuss priority students.

#2   Discuss new referrals.

#3   Identify students to receive $1.00 school store coupon.

#4   Other BEP issues or students.

FIGURE 5.4. Sample behavior support team meeting agenda for BEP.

tion should be presented to the behavior support team prior to implementing the BEP. In order for the BEP modifications to be effective, it is recommended that someone on the behavior support team be an expert in functional behavioral assessment (FBA). The adaptations to the BEP are based on the function of problem behavior, so having a person on the team who has experience with function-based behavior support will provide the team with the leadership that is needed to develop a more effective, modified BEP.

Training

The team responsible for managing the BEP intervention (whether it is the schoolwide positive behavior support team or the individual student service team, etc.) should receive training on their role in managing and supervising BEP implementation and on using data for decision making. For example, behavior teams will need to know how to use data to assess the effectiveness of the BEP. ODR data, BEP graphs, attendance records, and academic performance data can all be useful data sources.

Behavior teams should meet at least twice-monthly to examine student progress on the BEP. Team members will determine whether each student is making adequate progress and the program should be continued, whether modifications are needed, and/or whether a student is ready to be faded from the program. We have found it helpful to provide teams with case examples of DPRs and other data and ask them to practice making data-based decisions prior to implementing an actual BEP intervention. One of the primary mistakes made by BEP teams is ignoring the importance of a student's academic data. School teams should establish a process of examining behavior data (such as percentage of points on DPRs) alongside academic data (such as formative assessments like Curriculum-Based Measurement [CBM; Shinn, 1989] or Dynamic Indicators of Basic Early Literacy Skills [DIBELS; Good & Kaminski, 2001]). Other relevant academic data includes work completion rates and quarterly grades.

More information on using data for decision making is presented in Chapter 7.

ADMINISTRATOR

Roles and Responsibilities

The administrator plays a key role in developing and implementing the BEP. He or she must agree to allocate resources to the intervention prior to implementation and is critical in helping solicit commitment from the faculty for the program. It is often easier for staff to commit to participation if the administrator believes in the prevention philosophy of the BEP intervention and has a good rapport with the faculty. If the administrator has a reputation of bringing new programs and interventions to the school every year and has not supported implementation of these interventions, the faculty will see the BEP as the new "intervention for the year" and will be skeptical about whether it will be sustained. In contrast, if the administrator has effectively committed to systems change efforts such as implementing a schoolwide discipline plan, the faculty likely have experienced success with prevention. It is important for the administrator to communicate that the BEP is not an "intervention of the year" but rather a system that will be implemented to support students at risk year after year.

Once the administrator has helped develop faculty support and has committed resources to the BEP, he or she remains involved in helping the team match the BEP intervention with the school culture. *The administrator should attend the professional development day used for BEP development and implementation.* Some schools have tried to develop the BEP without administrator involvement, but many decisions such as allocation of space, meeting times, and staff training cannot be made without the administrator present. If the administrator is unable to be present during the professional development day, the day should be rescheduled to ensure the BEP is designed appropriately.

After BEP development and implementation, the administrator should attend behavior support team meetings at least twice a month. By staying involved, the administrator remains aware of student progress, or lack thereof, and may be assigned administrator-specific responsibilities.

The final, and crucial, role that the administrator must serve is as the implementation leader in the school building. The administrator's job is to provide feedback to teachers who are not implementing the BEP correctly. Some teachers may be too harsh and consistently give students low scores on the BEP. Other teachers may write negative comments on the DPR. Some teachers may not provide feedback on a regular basis to the student. Because the BEP coordinator is typically an educational assistant, it is inappropriate to expect this person to give corrective feedback to teachers. In addition to providing corrective feedback, the administrator should also provide reinforcement and positive comments to teachers who are doing a good job implementing the BEP. We have found it helpful to provide administrators with an overview of the critical features of the BEP and a list of their roles/responsibilities, which are detailed in Figure 5.5

TEACHING STAFF

Roles and Responsibilities

Prior to voting on whether or not to support the BEP, teachers should be informed about their classroom-based BEP responsibilities. Teachers are expected to greet the student positively at the beginning of the school day (for elementary school) or each class period (for middle and high school). The teacher is responsible for providing feedback on the DPR at predetermined times. It is impractical to expect the student to remember to regularly request feedback from the teacher, especially in the elementary school grades. *It is the teacher's responsibility to remember to provide feedback at the end of each period or transition and to provide an explanation for the rating that the student earned.* Older students can help teachers remember to provide feedback, but ultimately the responsibility lies with the teacher who is implementing the intervention. Sample feedback statements are listed in Figure 5.6. Each feedback period is a teaching opportunity. Teachers use these opportunities to provide positive examples of appropriate behavior (e.g., "Raising your hand was an example of being respectful") and negative examples (e.g., "Grabbing a pencil from Juanita was not an example of keeping your hands and feet to yourself"). During the feedback, teachers should also prompt for appropriate behavior (e.g., "Tomorrow let's work on. . . . ") and reinforce the student for following expectations, or making improvements in behavior.

What is the BEP?
- BEP is a check-in, check-out intervention implemented with students who are at risk for, but not currently engaging in, serious problem behavior.
- It should be one of the many secondary level/Tier II behavior interventions in your school to support students at risk.

Is my school ready to implement the BEP?
- Please refer to the BEP readiness checklist to determine if your school is in a good position to implement this intervention with fidelity.

What are the resources needed to implement the intervention?
- 10–15 hours per week paraprofessional time for check-in, check-out, and data management.
- Half- to full-day BEP development time for behavior support team.
- Allocate 20 minutes at least twice per month for reviewing BEP data in team meetings.
- Money required for reinforcers, NCR paper, follow-up training, etc.

What is my role as an administrator?
- Be involved with the team that develops the BEP to fit the culture of your school.
- Serve on the team that analyzes BEP data for decision making.
- *CRITICAL*: Provide feedback/coaching to teachers who are not implementing the BEP with fidelity or are being too harsh/negative.
- Give the BEP a high profile in the school.
  - Reinforce teachers for good implementation.
  - Reinforce students for doing well on the intervention.
  - Be involved in updates to staff on how the intervention is working.

FIGURE 5.5. BEP overview for administrators.

The following are suggestions for giving corrective feedback to the student on his or her DPR. Remember to focus and pay attention to the behavior you want to see more of, but let the student know why he or she received the score you gave him or her. Stay positive and upbeat and try to avoid being critical or sarcastic.

For best possible scores:
Wow, you got all [almost all] 2's today! You kept your hands and feet to yourself, and you followed directions. I liked the way you asked nicely for your book from Ashley. Way to go!

For good scores:
_____ [student name], you are doing so well! Look at that score! I saw that you kept your hands to yourself while you were working on that poster. You're going to make your goal! I saw you trying very hard today to stick to the rules and make your goal. Even though you got some 1's today because you were talking instead of doing your work, you did really well on keeping your hands, feet, and other objects to yourself.

For low scores:
Looks like you were having some trouble today. I know you can follow all the rules and finish your work but I didn't see you doing that today. Throwing your book is not keeping objects to yourself and its important not to use unkind words. What do you think you'll work on tomorrow? You've had some really good days, so even though you missed your goal today, because of being out of your seat and not completing your work, I know you can do much better.

FIGURE 5.6. Sample handout: Things to Say to Keep Students Motivated.

Teachers are also expected to make referrals to the behavior support team if they believe a student could benefit from the BEP or another intervention. Teachers should be informed of the preventative nature of Tier II interventions like the BEP. They should be encouraged to make a referral when students are just beginning to act out rather than waiting until problem behavior has escalated. Once a student has been referred and determined appropriate for the BEP, the teacher will need to collect 3–5 days of baseline data before the student begins the intervention. In terms of the day-to-day operations of the BEP, teachers are asked to provide feedback to the behavior support team on how the intervention is going. This feedback can include information about how the student is responding, a request for additional training on the intervention, or providing the behavior support team with information that may explain performance on the BEP.

Training

Initial Teacher Training

After staff have voted and agreed to implement the BEP intervention, they will need training on how to implement the intervention with individual students in their classroom. They will also need to know general information about how to make a referral and how students will be faded from the intervention over time. Figure 5.7 outlines both the training content and the materials that will be needed for this all-staff training. This information should be presented at the beginning of the school year after the staff has committed to the intervention. It can be used again if additional training sessions become necessary. Each new school year brings new school staff, so this training should be available on an annual basis.

Training the entire staff on the BEP intervention typically occurs during a regularly scheduled staff meeting. We have found that if training materials are well organized and if the staff have already received background information on the BEP, the training can occur during 30–40 minutes of a regularly scheduled staff meeting. During the training, all of the school's staff will

Training content
- Characteristics of students who are good candidates for the BEP
- How to make a referral
- How to complete the DPR
- How to provide motivating feedback
- Basic information about fading students off the BEP
- How students are rewarded on the program
- Frequently asked questions regarding BEP implementation

Materials needed
- DPR (on PowerPoint or overhead)
- Referral form (on PowerPoint or overhead)
- Consent form (on PowerPoint or overhead)
- Things to Say to Keep Students Motivated (handout)
- Frequently Asked Questions (handout)

FIGURE 5.7. BEP staff training.

need to be given information on what type of students are good candidates for the BEP and how to make a referral. Information regarding which students are appropriate or inappropriate, such as that provided in Table 3.1, is useful to include during the training. In addition, staff should be shown a copy of the school's parent consent form, as they will likely be involved in helping to get consent for the intervention.

All staff should also receive training on how to complete the DPR. This training should include examples of how to provide motivating feedback to students. Some schools provide role-play opportunities so that teachers can practice providing feedback and can demonstrate positive and negative examples of what feedback should sound like. It is important for staff to know that the feedback sessions should be quick, corrective (as needed), positive, and encouraging. Examples of motivating feedback were included in Figure 5.6.

It is important to provide staff training on the principle that the BEP is a time-limited intervention. After a student has demonstrated persistent improvement, the student should be faded off the intervention. Your school may choose to set a specific amount of time that each student participates in the BEP before data are examined and fading off the intervention is considered. Many schools that are not overwhelmed by a high number of students needing the BEP choose to use the end of the school year as a natural fade. The process of how students exit and graduate from the BEP should be explained to all school staff during the initial training. Staff should understand that when students meet their goals they will earn rewards or reinforcers. The initial training does not have to provide detailed reinforcement procedures, but rather can provide general information about how and when students will be reinforced.

During the initial training, we provide school staff with a handout about the frequently asked questions for BEP implementation. This document can be placed in the school's student handbook or in the teachers' positive behavior support binder. A sample handout addressing frequently asked questions is included in Figure 5.8.

Ongoing Teaching Training, Coaching, and Feedback

Several months may pass between the initial all-staff training and a teacher referral. As a result, teachers may benefit from a refresher on components of the intervention, how to greet the student, where the student should place his or her DPR, how to embed DPR ratings into their classroom routine, and additional practice on how to provide feedback.

Collection of baseline data should be emphasized in the refresher sessions. Depending on your school, it is recommended that 3–5 days of baseline data are taken to help with goal setting. Baseline data can also provide the teacher with practice implementing some of the components of the intervention.

Ongoing training and feedback provides teachers the opportunity to ask remaining questions about implementing the BEP and to address any concerns about the intervention. Awareness of teacher concerns will allow the behavior support team to address them prior to collaborating with individual teachers to implement the BEP. Some schools provide teachers with an additional handout at this point. The handout provides specific information about the BEP implementation process. This handout should be used after a teacher referral has been accepted, and while the referring teacher is preparing to implement the BEP intervention. A sample handout for supplemental teacher training information is provided in Figure 5.9.

The BEP is a schoolwide, check-in, check-out intervention program for students who are starting to engage in frequent problem behavior. The program will serve up to 30 students at a time. The goal of the BEP is to respond early to students who are acting out and to provide them with more frequent feedback on their behavior to prevent future problem behavior. Below are answers to some frequently asked questions about the BEP.

Which students would do well on the BEP?

Students who are starting to act out frequently but who are not currently engaging in dangerous (e.g., extreme aggression, property destruction) or severely disruptive (e.g., extreme noncompliance/defiance) behavior would be good candidates for the program. Students who engage in problem behavior across the day are good candidates for the program as opposed to students who have trouble only in one or two settings.

How do teachers participate in the BEP?

Teachers participate by providing both verbal and written feedback to students at predetermined times (see Daily Progress Report). The feedback should be quick, positive, and help remind the student what he or she needs to work on if the goal was not met. A sample feedback statement is "You did a nice job completing your work so you receive a '2' for work completion. I had to remind you not to flick Savannah's ponytail, so you got a '1' for keeping hands, feet, and other objects to yourself."

Who will be responsible for checking students in and out?

The BEP coordinator _____ [include name] will be in charge of checking students in and out. The coordinator will also keep track of the daily points earned and chart the progress for each student.

How do teachers make a referral?

A referral is made to the behavior support team of the school. In collaboration with the teacher, the team will determine whether the BEP is appropriate or whether another intervention would be more appropriate. The team will respond and provide feedback to the teacher within _____ [number] school days.

How long do students remain on the program?

At the end of every trimester, the behavior support team will look at each student's data to determine if he or she is ready to be faded off the BEP. Since there are a limited number of students (up to 30) who can receive the intervention, it will be important to fade students off as they become more independent in managing their own behavior.

FIGURE 5.8. Sample handout: Frequently Asked Questions.

Some teachers will continue to need ongoing support and feedback to successfully implement the BEP. Sometimes a member of the behavior support team needs to remind the teacher that he or she must provide feedback at predetermined times rather that at the end of the day. Other times, additional training and feedback is needed when teachers use the DPR to be punitive with students. Behavior support teams should consider retraining and feedback when the teacher consistently provides the lowest rankings, writes negative comments on the DPR (e.g., "Student was a jerk this period" or "Never on task!"), or regularly fails to complete the DPR. During these situations, it is critical for the *administrator* to provide the feedback and coaching to the teacher, as this is a work performance issue.

At the beginning of class
- The student brings his or her DPR to each class, and gives it to you (the teacher) to score during class.
- If the student doesn't give you the DPR right away (this may happen when he or she is just starting on the program), you may have to ask him or her for it.
- Be sure to be cheerful and positive with the student.
- Start out by setting the expectation for appropriate behavior. For example, you might say, "Thanks for giving me your Daily Progress Report—looks like you're all set to go! Remember to work on being responsible, safe, and kind." Or, if yesterday was a good class for the student you may say, "You're having a great week—keep it up! Keep trying to be an active learner who keeps hands and feet to self."
- Avoid negatives: Avoid saying things like "You're way behind—you're not going to make it" or "I don't want to see you doing anything like you did yesterday. . . . " Such comments will focus the student's attention on what not to do and you want to emphasize the appropriate, expected behavior. Let the student know you will be watching for him or her to follow expectations and engage in appropriate behavior.

How to score the DPR
- The DPR is quick and easy to score. The numbers on the DPR represent how well the student met behavioral expectations.
- The teacher will circle the highest number on the DPR if the student meets the expectation. For example, if the expectation was "Keep your hands, feet, and other objects to yourself," and the student was able to sit and move about the room without annoying other students, the teacher will circle the highest numbered rating.
- Circle the middle rating if the student had brief incidents of inappropriate behavior and had been warned twice (individually), but then repeated an incident of the behavior. For example, a student grabs another student's eraser without asking, causing a minor disruption *after you have already warned the student twice to keep his or her hands to him- or herself. Corrective feedback to the student may be (in a calm voice) "Allison, taking Eric's eraser is not keeping your hands to yourself as I asked you to do" and Alison receives a lower number on her DPR for the time period.*
- Circle the lowest number when the student did not meet the expectation. Students receiving this score have *repeated instances* (e.g., three) of not following directions, being off-task repeatedly, or doing something more serious such as fighting.

At the end of the time period:
- This is the time to show the student his or her scores and give him or her feedback on his or her behavior during class.
- Use phrases such as "Given you behavior . . . you earned . . ." versus "I am going to give you" as this puts the ownership of the behavior on the student.
- Spend just a minute or so with the student—it should not be a lengthy process.
- Whether their behavior has been good or poor, it is best to be specific about your feedback and again stay positive and cheerful.

For "best possible scores" (appropriate behavior)
- Be enthusiastic! Tell the student what he or she did to receive the rating and encourage him or her to continue. For example: "Wow! I am so proud of the way you followed directions, stayed on task, and were kind to your classmates. Looks like you'll make your goal!"

For "not so good" and "poor" ratings:
- These also need explanation. Keep the discussion upbeat and positive, but give specific feedback on what the student did or did not do during the class to meet expectations.
- Try not to criticize, use threats, or get into long explanations. Your rating is the final rating. For example: "Looks like you had a rough time listening and following directions today, but I know you can do it, I look forward to seeing you succeed tomorrow."

At the end of the day:
- The students take their DPRs with them when they leave class and they return the form to the BEP coordinator at the end of the day. The coordinator gives a copy to the student to take home for parent signature.

FIGURE 5.9. Sample handout: Additional BEP Training Information for Teachers.

Booster Training

Once or twice per year it is helpful to provide staff with booster training on how to implement the BEP and to problem-solve any schoolwide issues related to BEP implementation. Typically these trainings can be done during 10–20 minutes of a regularly scheduled school staff meeting. We have found that sharing the data with the staff on how the BEP is working is a great way to start these booster training sessions. Letting staff know how many students have been served, the amount of progress that has been made, and any other anecdotal information supporting the BEP helps start these trainings off on a positive note. Staff may need to be reminded about the characteristics of students who are appropriate for the BEP, how to make a referral, and any other issues that should be addressed during booster sessions.

Occasionally, a teacher who has experienced success with the BEP will want to use the intervention with every student engaging in behavior problems. During the booster training sessions, it is important to remind staff that the BEP is only one type of Tier II intervention and is not appropriate for all students. The staff may also want to review the other types of Tier II interventions that are available in their school. Booster sessions provide an additional opportunity for staff to ask questions about how to implement the BEP and to problem-solve any issues that have come up during implementation.

STUDENTS

Roles and Responsibilities

Participating students must understand the purpose of the BEP intervention and receive training on how to engage in the intervention. If the student remains unclear about the expectations for involvement, additional training should occur. Students are responsible for checking in with the BEP coordinator in the morning and checking out in the afternoon. Students pick up a new DPR every morning at check-in. Although teachers are responsible for providing students with feedback, students should hand the DPR to their teacher at the beginning of the school day (for elementary school) or at the beginning of each class period (for middle and high school). On occasion, students may need to remind their teachers to provide feedback.

Students are responsible for obtaining a new DPR from the BEP coordinator if they lose one during the school day. They must return the completed DPR to the BEP coordinator at check-out. Students are also responsible for taking home the DPR copy for parent feedback and taking it back the next day.

The primary responsibility for students on the BEP is to take ownership of their behavior. It is easy to receive positive feedback from teachers, but students on the BEP must also accept, and learn from, corrective feedback. Many students with problem behavior want to blame others for their behavioral challenges. An important objective of the BEP is that students will learn to self-manage their own behavior. Self-management begins with accepting responsibility for one's behavior.

If a teacher is giving unnecessarily harsh or punishing feedback, it is the student's responsibility to communicate this information to the BEP coordinator. The student's concern should be discussed at the behavior support team meeting. If the information is accurate, the administrator may need to step in to provide feedback to the teacher.

Training

Before a student begins the BEP intervention, it is critical to ascertain that he or she understands how to participate in all steps of intervention. First, the student is given an explanation for why he or she was selected for the intervention. Next, the purpose of the intervention is described. Students should understand that the BEP is a positive support system and that the goal is to support students to be more successful in schools. The BEP should *not* be introduced as a punishment for a student engaging in problem behavior.

Students should be informed that the BEP is a time-limited intervention and that, over time, the student will learn to manage his or her own behavior. The BEP helps the student learn which behaviors are positive examples of following expectations and which behaviors are negative examples. As soon as the student is fluent in meeting behavioral expectations, BEP support will be gradually faded.

Training of students on the BEP intervention is typically conducted by the BEP coordinator or by the counselor or school psychologist who supervises the BEP coordinator. The initial training takes 15–30 minutes, depending on the level of understanding of the student. Younger students may need more feedback and coaching on how to participate in the BEP. A summary of the topics that should be covered during the initial student training is included in Figure 5.10.

The logistics of participating in the BEP intervention are a major emphasis of the student training. Students need to know where and when to check in and where and when to check out. Many of the students who are appropriate candidates for the BEP find it challenging to accept corrective feedback from teachers. Furthermore, some of the younger students have a difficult time when they do not meet their daily point goals. For example, a young student might drop to the floor and have a tantrum if he or she does not earn enough points to receive a reinforcer for the day. The BEP coordinator should demonstrate how to appropriately respond to corrective feedback. Figure 5.2 provided information on one way to teach this skill to elementary school students.

- Purpose of the BEP intervention
  - Positive support system
  - Time-limited
  - Goal is to self-manage behavior
- Where and what time to check in
- Behavioral expectations and daily point goals
- Entering class and handing the DPR to teacher
- Getting feedback from teachers on the DPR
  - Role-play positive and negative examples of following expectations
- Where and when to check out
- Reinforcement system
  - What happens when daily point goals are met?
  - How to handle disappointment if goal is not met
- How to accept corrective feedback
- Plan for fading
  - Discuss BEP graduation and alumni parties

FIGURE 5.10. Topics for initial training of students on the BEP.

PARENTS

Roles and Responsibilities

Parents/guardians are responsible for signing the consent form to agree that their child may participate in the BEP intervention. This consent form outlines basic information about the intervention. The form also provides details regarding the parents' role in implementing the BEP intervention.

Parents are responsible for reviewing the DPR on a daily basis, providing feedback to their child, and signing the DPR. The student returns the DPR to the BEP coordinator on the following school day. If their child comes home without a DPR, the parents should first ask the child where it is. If the DPR cannot be found, and this happens two or more times in one week, the parents should call the school and determine the reason. Sometimes, students will hide or "lose" the DPR if they had a rough day and did not meet their goal. Parent should encourage their child to talk with them about both good days and difficult days. It is important for parents to try to help their children problem-solve ways to improve their behavior.

In some cases, parents are not home in the evenings to sign the DPR and provide feedback. In these cases, school staff should work with the parents to determine the best way to receive feedback from home. A grandparent, daycare provider, or responsible older sibling could provide feedback in place of a parent. Alternatively, if there is no one at home available to sign and provide feedback on a daily basis, a "surrogate parent" can be designated at school to provide the student with additional feedback and reinforcement. This surrogate parent might be a school counselor, office staff person, volunteer, or educational assistant.

Although it is not a required part of the intervention, we have seen students make greater behavioral progress when parents provide additional reinforcement at home for meeting their daily point goal. Examples include 15 minutes of additional time to use the phone, watch TV, or stay up later. Parents should not remove privileges if their child does not meet his or her daily goal. Students who are at risk for problem behavior already receive frequent negative consequences throughout the day. The focus of the BEP intervention, however, is to provide more positive experiences and feedback for the student.

Finally, parents are responsible for communicating regularly with the school regarding their child's progress, or any other issues that may affect progress on the intervention. For example, if the student is having difficulty at home, has had lots of disruption in his or her home life, or perhaps has had a change in medication that impacts his or her behavior, this important information needs to be communicated to the school.

Oftentimes, a decline in progress on the BEP corresponds with challenges the student is experiencing at home. Regular communication between the parents and the school helps the behavior support team decide if the student should remain on the BEP until issues at home become less disruptive or if a different intervention/support is warranted.

Training

Parents should receive training on the purpose of the BEP, the expectations for their child, and the expectations for themselves. A list of important topics to cover during the parent BEP training is provided in Figure 5.11. Optimally, parents will come to the school for a 20–30 minute meeting with the BEP coordinator and the counselor or school psychologist. The student

- Purpose of the BEP intervention
  - Positive support system
  - Time-limited
  - Primary goal is to learn to self-manage behavior
- Expectations for their child's daily participation in the BEP
  - Check-in, teacher feedback, check-out, reinforcement system, home component
- Reviewing and signing the DPR
  - Focus on positive
  - Examples and nonexamples of feedback
- Providing additional reinforcement at home for meeting daily point goals
  - No negative consequences for failing to meet daily point goal
- Plan for fading
  - Discuss BEP graduation and alumni parties
- Troubleshooting and frequently asked questions
  - What to do if the student fails to bring the DPR home
  - Is my child being singled out as "bad child"?
  - Address any other questions or concerns

FIGURE 5.11. Training of parents on the BEP.

can receive training for the BEP at the same time that his parents are trained. It is not always possible for parents to meet with school staff prior to BEP implementation. Many parents are unable to take time off of work to come to the school. In these cases, parents' BEP training can occur by arranging for a phone meeting.

When working with parents, the trainer should emphasize the positive and time-limited nature of the program. Parents should learn that the primary objective of the BEP is to teach the student to successfully manage his or her own behavior. Parents need to know what is expected of their child throughout the day. They should be told to sign the DPR every day when the child returns home and to make sure that their child returns it to school the next day.

Parents should be encouraged to write positive or neutral comments on the DPR before returning it to school. The trainer must emphasize that parents should not punish the child on days when the point goal is missed. If punishment occurs, the student will soon start to avoid bringing the DPR home. Instead, encourage parents to generate a list of activities that can be earned at home for meeting daily point goals. Students can earn extra TV time, time with friends, time reading with parents, extra computer time, or a special game with their parents if they meet their daily point goals. At the end of the BEP parent training, parents should be encouraged to ask questions about any of the information covered in the training.

CHAPTER 6

Designing the BEP to Fit Your School

The BEP intervention is comprised of certain critical features that must always be in place. These features include the use of a DPR, a uniform implementation process across participating students, regular behavioral feedback to students, and frequent use of effective reinforcement. After ensuring that these critical features are in place, each behavior support team has some flexibility to design the BEP to fit well with their student population and school. The flexible features of the BEP include (1) designing DPRs; (2) naming the intervention to match the culture of the school; and (3) creating an effective reinforcement system. This chapter provides examples of how different schools have personalized their own BEP intervention.

DESIGNING A DPR

Determining Expectations

One of the behavior support team's first tasks is to design the school's DPR. In collaboration with the staff, the team decides which behavioral expectations will be listed on the DPR. Behavioral expectations should be positively worded. That is, expectations should describe the behavior that students are expected to perform rather than the behavior that they are expected to avoid. For example, positively stated expectations include "Follow directions the first time" or "Keep hands, feet, and objects to yourself." In contrast, negatively worded expectations include "No hitting," "No talking back," or "No disrespectful language."

We recommend that the behavior support team choose to use the school's Tier I (schoolwide) behavior expectations for the DPR expectations. Students who benefit from BEP support need more practice and feedback on the schoolwide expectations. Some school personnel disagree with this recommendation and assert that each student needs individualized goals. However, *use of individualized student goals considerably decreases the efficiency of the BEP.* The BEP coordinator manages check-in and check-out for up to 30 students. If each student has individual goals, the amount of time required to complete check-in and check-out increases dramatically. In addition, one reason that teachers can rapidly build fluency in implementing the BEP is that the DPR is similar across students. Once a teacher has supported one student on the BEP, he or she is easily able to implement the BEP with a second or third student. Individualized goals reduce the intervention's generalizability to new students. Finally, individualized goals increase the cost of the intervention. Rather than having one version of the DPR on NCR paper, each student would require copies of his individualized DPR on NCR paper.

We recommend using individualized goals only when a student consistently fails to make progress on the intervention. Use of individualized goals is then considered a BEP modification. A discussion of how and when to use BEP modifications is presented in Chapter 8.

As a compromise between using individualized goals or using schoolwide expectations, some schools list their schoolwide expectations, but allow space on the DPR for one individual goal for each student. If schools choose to use one individualized goal per student, we strongly recommend that the *student* write down the goal each morning, rather than require the *BEP coordinator* to complete this extra step. This saves time for the coordinator while increasing responsibility for the student.

Figure 6.1 illustrates a middle school DPR that includes space for an individualized goal. The schoolwide expectations are listed across the top of the DPR: "Be Respectful," "Be Responsible," and "Be Safe." Under the student's name is a place for the student to write in his or her individual goal. Next to the schoolwide expectations is a column marked "My Goal," which is used to rate the student's behavior in regard to his or her individualized goal. Individualized

Name: Chase Johnson   Date: 10/12/09

My Goal: Keep Hands and Feet to Myself

Parent Signature: Sylvia Johnson

0 = No 1 = Good 2 = Excellent	Be Respectful	Be Responsible	Be Safe	My Goal: Keep Hands and Feet to Myself	Teacher Initials	WOW!!! Comments
Period 1	② 1 0	② 1 0	② 1 0	② 1 0	AC	Way to Go!
Period 2	2 ① 0	② 1 0	② 1 0	2 ① 0	BK	Let's work on this together.
Period 3	② 1 0	② 1 0	② 1 0	2 ① 0	LS	
Period 4	2 1 ⓪	2 1 ⓪	2 ① 0	2 ① 0	CT	You can do better tomorrow!
Period 5	② 1 0	② 1 0	② 1 0	2 ① 0	TL	
Period 6	2 ① 0	② 1 0	② 1 0	② 1 0	SM	
Period 7	② 1 0	② 1 0	② 1 0	② 1 0	GN	Good Day!
Total	10	12	13	10	Total:	Total Percent: 80%

FIGURE 6.1. Example of a middle school DPR with an individualized goal.

Date: 11/3/09 _____   Student: Erika Young _____

0 = No	1= Good	2= Excellent

	Be Safe	**Be Respectful**	**Be Your Personal Best**		
	Keep hands, feet, and objects to self	Use kind words and actions	Follow directions	Work in class	Teacher initials
9:00–A.M. Recess	0 1 ②	0 1 ②	0 1 ②	0 ① 2	DS
A.M. Recess–Lunch	0 1 ②	0 1 ②	0 ① 2	0 1 ②	DS
Lunch–P.M. Recess	0 1 ②	0 ① 2	0 1 ②	0 1 ②	DS
P.M. Recess–3:40	0 1 ②	0 1 ②	0 1 ②	0 1 ②	DS
Total Points = 29 Points Possible = 32		Today 91 %		Goal 80 %	

Parent Signature: I. Young _____

WOW: I'm proud of you. _____

FIGURE 6.2. Example of an elementary school DPR with expectations defined.

goals should be short, easy to remember, and positively stated. There should be no more than five total expectations listed on the DPR. Requiring a feedback rating for more than five expectations is too cumbersome for teachers to easily embed into their classroom routine.

Some schools choose to further define schoolwide expectations by including examples on the DPR of how to follow those expectations. For example, if the schoolwide expectation is "Be Respectful," the definition on the DPR could read "Use kind words and actions." An example of this type of DPR is included in Figure 6.2. The schoolwide expectations "Be Safe," "Be Respectful," and "Be Your Personal Best" are further defined in the column subheadings. We have found that if schools are thorough and systematic in teaching the entire student population how to follow schoolwide expectations (including demonstrations of positive and negative behavioral examples), then adding additional details on the DPR is generally not necessary.

DPR Rating System

The DPR developed for your school should be teacher-friendly. In order to keep the BEP efficient, and thus manageable, DPRs should utilize numerical ratings of behavior, rather than require time-consuming narrative explanations. The DPRs illustrated in Figures 6.1 and 6.2 include a section for teacher comments. *It is not required that teachers complete these sections.* Instead, teachers are encouraged to provide written positive feedback when possible. In Figure

6.1, the column is labeled "WOW!!! Comments," prompting teachers to write positive, rather than negative, comments.

Students should receive lower ratings on their DPR if they are engaging in inappropriate behavior, but writing negative comments should not be allowed. By virtue of their behavior status, these students often receive negative corrective feedback throughout the day. We recommend the term "comments" not be used alone on the DPR. Instead, a word or phrase that encourages teachers to provide additional positive feedback should be inserted. Terms such as "WOW," "Successes," or "Celebrations" are good examples that prompt teachers to provide positive feedback.

Each DPR should include a range of scores. Some schools prefer to use a "0, 1, 2," ranking system, whereas other schools prefer to use "1, 2, 3." We recommend a 3-point (rather than 4- or 5-point) system, as this makes it easier to obtain consistent rankings across teachers. A key, defining the corresponding meaning of each numerical rating, should be included on the DPR. For example, in Figure 6.1 the DPR includes the following key: "0 = No" (the student did not meet the behavior expectation), "1 = Good" (the student did a good job meeting the expectations), and "2 = Great" (the student did a great job meeting the expectations).

Prior to implementation of the BEP, all school staff should clarify and agree on the difference between each rating. This will increase interrater reliability across teachers. In other words, if a student exhibits similar behavior in Classroom A and in Classroom B, then he or she should receive the same rating for that behavior from each teacher. If one teacher uses a much stricter standard for judging the student's behavior and the student consistently receives a "0" in the first classroom and a "2" in the second classroom for the same behavior, the student will become confused regarding what is appropriate and what is inappropriate. Teachers should be giving students consistent feedback about their behavior by providing consistently similar behavior ratings.

Schools might choose to adopt the following guidelines to increase interteacher rating consistency. If a student needs one reminder or correction during the period, he can still receive a "2." If the student needs two reminders or corrections, he receives a 1; three or more reminders equals a "0" ranking. This simple approach may or may not work for your school. Problem behavior is locally and contextually defined, so your school staff should agree on how to define each score on the ranking system.

Some schools list the definitions of each rating on the DPR. Figure 6.3 provides an example of a school that has a 4-point rating system, with the rating system key included on the DPR. We recommend that you attempt to keep the ratings key small enough so that the DPR fits on a half-page. This reduces the amount of expenditures related to copying costs and NCR paper.

The behavior support team must decide how many rating periods to include on the DPR. At a minimum, include four rating periods. Less than four precludes the student from having a difficult period/class, and still meeting his or her daily point goal. For middle and high school settings, the periods of the day are used as rating periods. If a school has six periods in a day, there will be six opportunities for the student to receive feedback on his or her behavior.

In elementary school settings, we recommend that the rating periods correspond to natural transitions in the school day. For example, as illustrated in Figure 6.2, a natural transition occurs before A.M. recess and before lunch. Optimally, the marking periods should not last longer than 75 minutes. Students on the BEP respond better when they receive feedback after short intervals of time. This is especially true for young children. However, if 75 minutes does

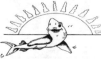

Shark Code

Sunset Elementary School

Checked in	YES	NO
Checked out	YES	NO
Parent Signature	YES	NO

Goal: 50%   55%   60%   65%   70%   75%   80%

Student: _____   Date: _____   M Tu W Th F   Goal: _____

Expectations	Arrival to Recess				Recess to Lunch				Lunch to Recess				Recess to Dismissal				Total
	Tough time	So-so	Good	Awe-some	Tough time	So-so	Good	Awe-some	Tough time	So-so	Good	Awe-some	Tough time	So-so	Good	Awe-some	
Safe	1	2	3	4	1	2	3	4	1	2	3	4	1	2	3	4	
Honest & Accountable	1	2	3	4	1	2	3	4	1	2	3	4	1	2	3	4	
Respectful & Kind	1	2	3	4	1	2	3	4	1	2	3	4	1	2	3	4	
Keep Practicing																	

Successes:

4 = Awesome: Met expectations with positive behavior; worked independently without any corrections/reminders
3 = Good: Met expectations with only 1 reminder/correction
2 = So-so: Needed 2–3 reminders/corrections
1 = Tough time: Needed 4 or more reminders/corrections

Parent/Guardian Signature: _____   **Note:** Parent comments can be included on the back of this form

FIGURE 6.3. Example of a DPR with a 4-point ranking system and ranking system defined.

not correspond with a natural transition, it is preferable to wait for a time when the teacher can easily incorporate student feedback into his or her classroom routine.

Some school teams have considered creating different DPRs to correspond with each different grade level. In response, we emphasize that increasing the number of DPR formats decreases the efficiency of the intervention. Elementary school teachers have argued that younger students (e.g., kindergarten and first grade) have different academic expectations and scheduling than older students (e.g., fourth, fifth, sixth grade). One school responded to this dilemma by creating two DPR formats, one for the lower grades and one for the upper grades.

Examples of the lower- and upper-grade DPRs are provided in Figures 6.4 and 6.5. In these examples, Vista Elementary School added an additional expectation of "Work Completion" to the three schoolwide expectations. The behavior support team felt it was important to include this additional expectation. Since they had only three schoolwide rules, adding an additional expectation did not make the rating system unmanageable for teachers. Prior to implementing this addition, they received feedback and approval from all staff in the school.

Nonclassroom Settings

Should nonclassroom settings be included on the DPR? Nonclassroom settings include places such as the lunchroom/cafeteria, playground, hallways, bus area, and bathrooms. The focus of the BEP intervention is on classroom behavior. Students who have problems only in unstructured settings, such as those listed above, should not be placed on the BEP intervention but rather should have an intervention that focuses on the setting where they are engaging in problem behavior. In most schools, there is not enough supervision on the playground or in cafeteria

**Vista Elementary ROAR Program
WILD CARD**

Name: _____   Date: _____

GOAL	9:05– A.M. Recess	A.M. Recess– Lunch	Lunch– P.M. Recess	P.M. Recess– 3:45
Follow directions the first time	0 1 2	0 1 2	0 1 2	0 1 2
Be on task	0 1 2	0 1 2	0 1 2	0 1 2
Keep hands, feet, and other objects to yourself	0 1 2	0 1 2	0 1 2	0 1 2
Work Completion	0 1 2	0 1 2	0 1 2	0 1 2

KEY
0 = No
1 = Somewhat . .
2 = YES!!

Successes: _____

Goal for Today: _____ %

Total for Today: _____ %

Teacher Signature _____   Parent Signature _____

FIGURE 6.4. Example of a lower elementary grade DPR.

**VISTA Elementary ROAR Program
WILD CARD**

Name: _____   Date: _____

GOAL	Reading	Language Arts	Spelling	Math	Science	Social Studies	Health
Follow directions the first time	0 1 2	0 1 2	0 1 2	0 1 2	0 1 2	0 1 2	0 1 2
Be on task	0 1 2	0 1 2	0 1 2	0 1 2	0 1 2	0 1 2	0 1 2
Keep hands, feet, and other objects to yourself	0 1 2	0 1 2	0 1 2	0 1 2	0 1 2	0 1 2	0 1 2
Work Completion	0 1 2	0 1 2	0 1 2	0 1 2	0 1 2	0 1 2	0 1 2

Teacher Initials   _____   _____   _____   _____   _____   _____   _____

KEY
0 = No
1 = Somewhat . .
2 = YES!!

Successes: _____   Assignments: _____

Goal for Today: _____ %

Total for Today: _____ %

Parent Signature _____

FIGURE 6.5. Example of an upper elementary grade DPR.

settings for up to 30 students to receive feedback at the same time. A playground supervisor could not effectively track the individual behavior of more than three to five students at a time. *We recommend that the DPR should not include nonclassroom settings.*

For a few students who have problem behavior in classroom settings, as well as during recess, we have had success in using a "recess contract" in combination with the DPR. The recess contract looks similar to the DPR (i.e., same behavioral expectations), but is kept separate from the DPR. It is rated by the person who is supervising the playground or other unstructured area. There should only be one or two students per recess who receive this type of feedback. Schools that utilize a recess contract typically employ a separate reinforcement system for it. Alternatively, with a little extra work on the part of the BEP coordinator, recess contract points could be embedded into the BEP overall daily point goal.

Other Considerations

BEP teams often choose to include a column on the DPR for teachers to initial their rating (illustrated in Figure 6.5). We also recommend providing a place for parent signature as well as space for parents to provide additional positive feedback to their child.

In designing the DPR, consider whether or not to include a section for the student's percentage point goal. To increase efficiency, many schools use the same goal across students (i.e., 80% or higher). However, in order to experience initial success on the BEP, some students will need to start at a lower percentage point goal. In Figure 6.3, there is a section for the students to use individualized goals by circling a goal between 50% and 80% of points. In addition to having a section for the percentage goal, there should be a section to write what the student's total points were for the day. This will allow parents to easily determine if the student has met his or her goal and will also ease the task of data entry for the BEP coordinator.

Some elementary schools have struggled with how to include nondaily activities on the DPR. For example, elementary students often attend physical education (PE), music, library, art, and computer lab one time per week. Many schools have combined those activities into one marking section. Rather than listing these rotations separately, they will list "PE/Music/CompLab" as one of the times in the day the students can receive feedback. Another issue to consider is early dismissal days. In order to provide adequate teacher preparation time, some schools have early dismissal once a week. In that case, it is important to include a section on the DPR that lists the total points possible for these early dismissal days. For example, an elementary school might have a total of 40 points possible on every day of the week except Friday. On early-dismissal Fridays, students could earn a total of 30 points. If students come to school late or need to leave early, the rating periods that were missed should be crossed out so that the BEP coordinator knows to not calculate those periods in the total score. *In other words, percentage of points should accurately reflect the total number of points possible on any given day.*

Summary

The following is a summary of recommendations for creating a DPR to fit your school:

- Include schoolwide expectations on the DPR.
- Expectations must be positively stated.

- No more than five expectations should be listed on the DPR.
- Use of DPR must be teacher-friendly and require teachers to circle ratings rather than provide narrative feedback.
- Need to include a narrow range of scores (e.g., "1, 2, 3").
- Include a ratings key on the DPR.
- Include a column for "successes" rather than just "comments."
- DPR should fit on half sheet of an 8½" × 11" piece of paper to reduce copying costs.
- Nonclassroom settings should *not* be included on the DPR.
- Include a column for teacher to initial rating and a line for parent signature and parent comments.
- Determine if the percentage point goal will be listed.
- Include an area for total points earned.

NAMING THE BEP INTERVENTION AND THE DPR

We encourage schools to rename the BEP and the DPR to fit the culture of their school. Many schools like to rename the BEP to match the mascot of their school. This choice can be left to the behavior support team. We recommend requesting input from all school staff when renaming the BEP and the DPR. Table 6.1 provides examples of alternative names for the BEP, some of which are based on different school mascots.

Why is renaming the program so important? It helps the staff of the school feel more personally connected to the intervention. Rather than adopting an intervention that was designed and implemented in another school, the BEP becomes an intervention that was redesigned to fit your school's demographics and characteristics. When renaming the intervention, it is important to focus on the positive nature of the BEP. The BEP should be a positive behavior support system and not a punishment system. Parents and students are more likely to engage in the intervention if its name indicates support rather than punishment. For example, renaming the BEP "Supporting Our Antisocial and Rowdy Students," or SOARS, would likely turn off parents, students, and teachers. In contrast, using the same acronym, the BEP could be renamed "Students On A Road 2 Success."

When renaming the BEP, we recommend that you do not use the terms "behavior support plan" or "behavior contract." To begin with, the BEP is not an *individualized* behavior support plan and it is critical that teachers not confuse this program with Tier III levels of behavior support. Students who need Tier III support require comprehensive functional behavioral assessments and individualized behavior support plans. In our experience, many teachers have tried behavior contracts in their classrooms. When they request assistance from the behavior support team, they are looking for an intervention beyond what has already been implemented to support the student. If the team mentions implementing a "behavior contract," the teacher might reply, "I've already tried that."

Choose a name that is easy to remember and teach. If you rename the BEP using an acronym such as "HAWK—Helping A Winning Kid," it is important that teachers, parents, and students know what the acronym means.

TABLE 6.1. Examples of Different Names for the BEP and the DPR

Mascot	Name of the intervention	Name of the DPR
	Behavior Education Program	Daily Progress Report
Eagles	Students On A Road 2 Success (SOARS) Program	SOARS Card
Skyhawks	Helping A Winning Kid (HAWK) Program	HAWK Report
	Hello, Update, and Goodbye (HUG) Program	HUG Card
Lions	Reinforcement of Appropriate Response (ROAR) Program	Wild Card
	Check and Connect Program	Check and Connect Card
Wildcats	Positive Action With Support (PAWS) Program	PAWS Card
Buffalos	Building Up Fantastic Futures *or* Be Up for Future Success (BUFF) Program	BUFF Card
Tigers	Trying All I can to Learn (TAIL) Program	Tiger Tail Card
Rams	Rams Achieve More (RAM) Program	RAM Card
Zebras	Heading with Energy in the Right Direction (HERD) Program	Earn Your Stripes Card
Eagles	Excel And Gain Life Educational Skills (EAGLES) Program	EAGLES Card
Sharks	Safe, Honest, Accountable, Responsible, and Kind (SHARK) Program	Shark Code

DEVELOPING AN EFFECTIVE
REINFORCEMENT SYSTEM FOR THE BEP

Rationale

Students who qualify for the BEP have been unsuccessful in meeting schoolwide behavioral expectations at the Tier I level of behavior support. These students typically need additional feedback and reinforcement in order to learn appropriate ways to meet schoolwide behavioral expectations. One goal of the BEP is to help the student build positive relationships with adults in the school. A second goal is to help the student become independent in managing his or her own behavior. To achieve independence, students should be gradually faded from the structured reinforcement system of the BEP to the informal reinforcement of the schoolwide behavior system.

The most powerful reinforcer in the BEP intervention should be the BEP coordinator. The BEP coordinator should be someone whom the students like, trust, and look forward to seeing on a daily basis. Some reinforcement systems that are developed by schools for use with the

BEP will include tangible items such as small toys or snacks. These tangible rewards should always be paired with social praise and acknowledgment from the BEP coordinator.

Assessing Reinforcer Preference

When the behavior support team develops the BEP to fit the culture of their school, there is some preliminary development of the reinforcement system. For example, the team typically determines the percentage of points that students must earn in order to receive a reinforcer. The team may also consider the different types of reinforcers that students can earn. It is important, particularly for middle or high school students, to choose rewards that are perceived as truly reinforcing by the students themselves.

A *positive reinforcer* is defined as an event or stimulus that follows some behavior and increases the likelihood that the behavior will occur again in the future (Alberto & Troutman, 2006). In other words, whether or not a reward is reinforcing is determined by its impact on the student's behavior, not by whether or not we expect it to have high value to the student. For example, we might consider extra time on the computer to be an effective (and relatively cheap) reinforcer for middle school students. However, if earning extra computer time is not desired by the student, and if it does not cause the student to continue to follow behavioral expectations, then it is not a reinforcer for that student. Indeed, for a student who struggles with keyboarding skills, extra computer time could actually be perceived as a punishment. The team determines whether or not a reward is reinforcing by examining its impact on the student's behavior. If, after receiving a reward for meeting his or her goal, the student continues to meet his or her goal or demonstrates an improvement in his or her behavior, the team can assume that they have chosen an effective reinforcer for that student.

School staff often choose "rewards" for students but in the end discover these rewards are not very reinforcing. That is, the rewards do not have the intended impact on the students' future behavior. As an example, one school provided school supplies (pencils, erasers, etc.) as rewards for students who met their daily point goal. Many of the students complained that they already had enough supplies and would be more interested in earning a snack or extra recess time. Once the school allowed the students to choose rewards for which they were willing to work (i.e., activities or items that were actually reinforcing), students' progress on the BEP improved.

One way to assess reinforcer preference is for students to complete a reinforcer checklist. (A sample copy of a reinforcer checklist is included in Figure 6.6 and Appendix E.1.) The reinforcer checklist is typically used to assess students' interest in earning different types of long-term reinforcers rather than daily reinforcers. It should be noted that this is just one example of different reinforcers that students may be interested in earning. We recommend that the behavior support team collaborate with school staff to generate a list of inexpensive or free reinforcers that are available in their school setting. Every school has teachers with certain talents they may be willing to share or special activities that are already a part of the schoolwide reward system that can be used with the BEP. For example, in one school we worked with a teacher who was a former semiprofessional soccer player. Students on the BEP could earn a one-on-one soccer lesson from this teacher for meeting their goals for a certain number of days. In another school, the janitor was willing to provide guitar lessons as a reinforcer for students receiving BEP support.

Reinforcer Checklist
(To be completed by the student)

Please circle YES or NO if the item or activity is something you would like to earn.

Activity Reinforcers

Video game	YES	(NO)		Basketball	YES	(NO)
Swimming	YES	(NO)		Magazine	(YES)	NO
Watching video/DVD	YES	(NO)		Drawing	(YES)	NO
Walking	YES	(NO)		Field trips	(YES)	NO
Comic books	(YES)	NO		Puzzles	(YES)	NO
Play-Doh	(YES)	NO		Board game	YES	(NO)
Craft activities	(YES)	NO		Card game	YES	(NO)

Please list any other favorite activities you would like to earn.

Computer Games
_____

Material Reinforcers

Stickers	(YES)	NO		Erasers	YES	(NO)
Special pencils	(YES)	NO		Bubbles	YES	(NO)
Lotions	YES	(NO)		Play-Doh	(YES)	NO
Colored pencils/crayons	(YES)	NO		Rings	YES	(NO)
Free tardy pass	YES	(NO)		Puzzles	(YES)	NO
Bookmarks	YES	(NO)		Trading cards	(YES)	NO
Action figures	YES	(NO)		Small toys	(YES)	NO
Free assignment pass	(YES)	NO		Necklaces	YES	(NO)

Please list any other favorite items you would like to earn.

_____

Edible Reinforcers

Small one-bite candies	(YES)	NO		Cereal	YES	(NO)
Larger candy	(YES)	NO		Fruit	YES	(NO)
Vending machine drink	YES	(NO)		Pretzels	(YES)	NO
Juice/punch	YES	(NO)		Potato chips	(YES)	NO
Vegetables and dip	YES	(NO)		Corn chips	YES	(NO)
Crackers	YES	(NO)		Cookies	(YES)	NO
Donuts	(YES)	NO		Bagels	YES	(NO)
Candy bars	(YES)	NO		Cheese	YES	(NO)

Please list any other favorite name brands or snacks you would like to earn.

Gum
_____

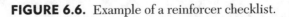

(cont.)

FIGURE 6.6. Example of a reinforcer checklist.

Social Reinforcers

Pat on the back	YES	NO		Verbal praise	YES	NO
Extra P.E./gym time	YES	NO		Free time	YES	NO
Games with teacher	YES	NO		Field trips	YES	NO
Games with friends	YES	NO		Special seat	YES	NO
Lunch with friends	YES	NO		High 5	YES	NO
Visit with friends	YES	NO		Awards	YES	NO

Please list any other favorites you would like to earn.

FIGURE 6.6. *(cont.)*

When possible, we recommend trying to identify reinforcers that involve spending time with others, particularly socially competent peers. Students who qualify for the BEP often have difficulty with peer relations and therefore will benefit from more positive interactions with peers through structured reinforcement activities. For example, some schools have allowed the student to choose four other students to participate with him or her in extra gym time earned for meeting daily point goals.

Reinforcers for Checking In and Checking Out

The primary reinforcer for students checking in and out should be the personal connection with the BEP coordinator. However, we have noticed that sometimes when students have a rough day and do not meet their daily point goal, they are less likely to check out at the end of the day. To increase the incentive for checking out some schools have instituted a "lottery system." Students receive a lottery ticket for checking in on time in the morning and receive a second lottery ticket for checking out at the end of the day. A sample copy of a school's lottery ticket is presented in Figure 6.7.

At the end of the week, a drawing is held for students on the BEP. The more times a student checks in and checks out, the more chances he or she has to win. The prizes for the drawings are small (e.g., coupon to school store or snack bar), but students typically enjoy this extra opportu-

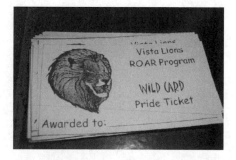

FIGURE 6.7. Sample lottery ticket from Vista Elementary.

nity to earn reinforcers. To make the drawing more exciting, some schools employ a "mystery motivator" format and allow the student to select from one of three potential prizes that are placed in sealed envelopes. To provide further reinforcement and encouragement, the weekly prizewinners' names are posted for other students on the BEP to see. This public posting should not be accessible to all students in the school as this could create issues related to other students wanting to be on the intervention.

Some of our schools feel it is unnecessary to have a lottery system because the students really enjoy participating in the program. The lottery system is a component that can be added if a school is experiencing problems with students consistently checking in and checking out. Your school may want to start without a lottery system and add it only if it becomes necessary.

Reinforcers for Meeting Daily Point Goals

For the BEP to be effective, students should receive reinforcement for meeting their daily point goals. One of the biggest mistakes schools make when first implementing the BEP is misunderstanding the importance of frequent reinforcement during the first 2 weeks of the intervention. If a student does not meet his or her goal within the first 2 weeks on the BEP, the goal is set too high. The student's interest in the BEP and willingness to actively participate will rapidly wane.

Collecting baseline data is critical to setting achievable daily point goals. For the sake of efficiency, we have recommended using the same daily point goal for all students. Occasionally, however, students will need a lower goal to achieve initial success. Baseline data will help identify these students.

One way to motivate students to achieve consistent success on the BEP is to reward the student for meeting his or her point goal for a specified number of days. Behavior support teams will often set a consecutive criterion (e.g., student must earn 80% of points on 5 *consecutive* school days) rather than a cumulative criterion (e.g., after a *total* of 5 school days of earning 80% of points, the student can earn the reinforcer). We recommend using a cumulative criterion. Students on the BEP will have difficult days and therefore a cumulative goal is more achievable and reinforcing than a consecutive goal.

Daily/Short-Term Reinforcers

Some type of small, daily reinforcement is often effective in maintaining students' consistent engagement in the intervention. Although we recommend avoiding the use of edible reinforcers, many schools have found that a piece of candy or a small snack is highly valued by students at the end of the day. We encourage schools to choose healthy snacks, if food is to be used as a reinforcer. While the use of daily reinforcers for meeting point goals is helpful, it is not required. The behavior support team should consider the cost of daily reinforcers and the financial resources budgeted for the BEP intervention.

One creative approach to daily reinforcers is the "Spin the Wheel" game. This game gives students a random chance of receiving one out of a variety of rewards. This approach to daily reinforcement is more effective in elementary school settings than in middle or high school settings. Figure 6.8 provides an example of a spinning wheel that was implemented in Vista Elementary School.

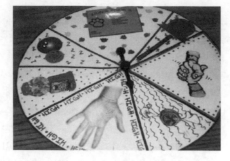

FIGURE 6.8. Spinner system for daily BEP rewards.

On the spinning wheel pictured in Figure 6.8, the wider sections of the wheel (and thus higher chances of winning) include social rewards such as a "high five" or a secret handshake. It is preferable for students to work for social reinforcement over tangible reinforcers. The narrower sections of the wheel (thus, lower chances of winning) include a piece of candy, a gumball, or a sticker. Two schoolwide rewards have been included on the wheel. One is a "Lion's Pride 5" ticket, which is a token used for schoolwide rewards. The other is a "Lion's Loot" dollar which goes back to the student's classroom to be put into a classroom bank. At this example school, the "dollar" is associated with a schoolwide social skills intervention. The student on the BEP has the chance to earn dollars for the entire class to engage in an activity.

Long-Term Reinforcers

Many schools provide opportunities for students on the BEP to earn long-term reinforcers. Long-term reinforcers typically require students to meet their daily point goal across several days or even several weeks. These rewards are typically identified using the reinforcer checklist as items individual students are interested in earning.

To manage a long-term reinforcer system, some schools use a "credit card" scheme to tally points. Other schools call this a "savings card" or "point card." Regardless of its name, the aim is to give the student a choice between using points to receive smaller reinforcers or saving points to earn larger, long-term reinforcers. The BEP credit card system allows students to earn more points for better performance on their DPR. Here is an example of how one school outlined points that students can earn:

- \> 70% on DPR = 1 point on credit card
- \> 80% on DPR = 2 points on credit card
- \> 90% on DPR = 3 points on credit card
- 100% on DPR = 4 points on credit card

Figure 6.9 illustrates an example of a BEP credit card developed by Vista Elementary School that has been used successfully in both elementary and secondary school settings.

The BEP coordinator (older students can self-manage this process) marks the number of points earned by the student by highlighting or placing a checkmark in each box. We recom-

1	2	3	4	5	6	7	8	9	10
X̶	X̶	X̶	X̶	X̶	X̶	X̶	X̶	X̶	X̶
X	X	X	X	X	X	X	X	X	X
									30
									40
									50
									60
									70
									80
									90
									100

FIGURE 6.9. Sample credit card.

mend against using a special stamp or hole-punch as it would be fairly time-consuming to do this for up to 30 students per day.

The credit card system requires that the school develop a menu of reinforcers with different point values. Once a student earns enough points for the reinforcer he or she desires, the points are exchanged with the BEP coordinator. The credit card is marked to show that the student has spent those points.

The credit card can be used until the student fills up a card with a hundred points. Then a new credit card is given to the student. In Figure 6.9, the student has earned a total of 20 points across 9 school days and has decided to exchange 10 points for 5 minutes of extra computer time to play games during lunch.

Who Provides the Reinforcement?

Typically, the BEP coordinator manages the BEP reinforcement system. If a student earns additional computer time, the BEP coordinator provides the time, or collaborates with one of the student's teachers to provide the time. Members of the behavior support team are also often involved in delivering reinforcement. School counselors and school psychologists typically have more flexibility in their day than teachers to provide time-based reinforcers such as extra gym time, extra computer time, or even an extra recess.

When designing the BEP to fit your school culture, the issue of how to manage the reinforcement system must be addressed. The BEP will be less effective if students do not receive reinforcement soon after they have earned it. Imagine if a student has earned basketball time, but the school counselor in unable to play basketball with the student until 3 weeks after the reinforcer is earned. Extended delays in delivery of reinforcement will result in student frustration and reduced commitment to the intervention.

Reinforcement for Teachers

Reinforcement for active and successful participation in the BEP intervention should not be limited to participating students. Teachers should receive reinforcement as well. Effective teacher participation is the backbone of an effective BEP intervention. Teachers must provide ratings of student behavior on a regular basis and ensure that the student understands how to meet the behavioral expectations.

Teachers complete the DPR on a daily basis but may not know how the student is progressing overall. One way to reinforce teacher participation is to share their student's DPR data graph with them. Additional strategies can be used to reward teachers for implementing the BEP with fidelity. Some schools encourage BEP students to nominate their teachers for a "Supportive Teacher BEP Award." Once a month, a different teacher is acknowledged based on student nomination. Other schools examine the positive teacher comments written on the DPR and recognize a teacher for being a positive participant in the BEP intervention. Whatever approach is chosen, it is important to recognize teachers' efforts and support in helping students achieve success on the BEP.

Reinforcer Budget

The behavior support team will likely have to grapple with the costs of reinforcers against the backdrop of budgetary constraints. School budgets are often tight, and the BEP should be implemented in a cost-effective manner. The greatest financial outlay is the expense of funding a BEP coordinator for approximately 10–15 hours a week. The costs of reinforcers should be a minor portion of the BEP budget. The following list provides recommendations for keeping expenses low, while still implementing an effective reinforcement system.

- Solicit donations from the community. All donations to a school are tax deductible, and the school can publicly acknowledge the business or community agency as a supporter of the school.
- Choose rewards that involve use of time rather than the purchase of tangible items. Some of our favorite examples include (1) time with a preferred adult; (2) time with a (socially competent) peer; (3) time to read a favorite comic book or novel; or (4) extra gym, recess, art, computer, or library time.
- Students will work to earn opportunities for leadership or other positions of status. These include (1) first in line for lunch; (2) leading the class in a lesson; (3) library helper; (4) computer helper; (5) broadcasting morning announcements; and (6) leading social skill lessons with the support of counselor.
- Students will work to avoid activities that the student perceives as aversive. With teacher permission, the following can be used as reinforcers: (1) one free homework; (2) one free assignment; (3) skipping problems on an assignment; or (4) being excused from homeroom to do a preferred activity.
- When purchasing games or toys, choose items that are reusable. Schools have purchased board games, remote-controlled cars, Game Boy, or Nintendo DS. All of these items involved an initial investment up front, but could be used over and over again.

Summary

The following is a summary of recommendations for developing reinforcement systems for the BEP:

- Assess student preference for long-term reinforcers.
- Use baseline data to assess if the standard daily point goal is appropriate for the student.
- Consider implementing an incentive system for checking in and checking out.
- Determine if there will be both short-term and long-term reinforcers.
- Identify a system to manage long-term rewards, such as the credit card system.
- Determine who will deliver the reinforcers. Avoid lengthy delays in reinforcer delivery as this results in frustration and reduced student commitment.
- Develop a system to provide reinforcement to teachers who actively support the BEP.

CHAPTER 7

Measuring Response
to the BEP Intervention and Fading

As discussed in Chapter 2, the BEP has been shown to be effective with the majority (50–75%) of students who receive the intervention. Schools interested in implementing the BEP should have assessment systems to document both the extent to which the BEP is implemented with fidelity (i.e., implemented as planned) and student response to the intervention. Once a student has demonstrated a continuous positive response to the BEP, the school should plan to begin to fade the student off the intervention. The purpose of this chapter is to discuss ways to measure fidelity, to determine response to intervention, and to set up procedures for fading the BEP.

MEASURING FIDELITY OF BEP IMPLEMENTATION

Prior to assessing whether students are responding to the BEP, schools should assess the extent to which they are implementing the BEP with fidelity. Some schools have poor outcomes for students receiving the BEP intervention, but upon further examination, it is determined that the critical features of the intervention are not firmly in place. The positive outcomes that have been documented in the research literature are related to high fidelity of implementation of the BEP by school staff. In general, we have seen that the parental participation component is typically the weakest element implemented (Hawken et al., 2007). Overall, however, studies have shown that school personnel can implement the BEP with high fidelity, that is, greater than 80% fidelity.

The School-Wide Evaluation Tool (SET; Horner et al., 2004) was designed to evaluate the extent to which schools have implemented Tier I or Tier II levels of positive behavior support. The SET involves a combination of interviews, observations, and review of permanent products to document a school's fidelity of implementation of their schoolwide discipline plan. The BEP Fidelity of Implementation Measure (BEP-FIM) was modeled after the SET and was designed to measure the extent to which schools are implementing the BEP with fidelity. A copy of the BEP-FIM is included in Appendix F.1. Although formal psychometric properties (e.g., reliability and validity) have not been established for the BEP-FIM, it is a tool for schools to document BEP implementation.

Some of the information from the BEP-FIM comes from the daily data gathered by the BEP coordinator on the BEP check-in, check-out form. Each day the BEP coordinator is recording whether students check in, check out, and meet their daily goal, and whether the DPR has come back signed from the parent/guardian. The other items on the BEP-FIM relate to whether (1) the school has allocated adequate resources to the BEP; (2) the administrator is an active participant; and (3) data are used for decision making.

MEASURING RESPONSE TO THE BEP INTERVENTION

Daily Progress Reports

The BEP has a built-in progress monitoring tool because the teachers complete the DPR on a daily basis. Each day, information is summarized to determine if the student has met his or her daily point goal. Data are summarized by percentage of points earned, and graphed on a regular basis to assess whether or not the student is regularly meeting goals. Prior to BEP implementation, the behavior support team must make some decisions regarding database management. The primary question to answer is which system will be used to summarize the data. Currently, most schools summarize data by using the School-Wide Information System–Check-In, Check-Out (SWIS-CICO) web-based system or by using a Microsoft Excel™ spreadsheet graphing program to create their own database.

The School-Wide Information System (SWIS) was originally designed to organize and summarize office discipline referrals (ODRs) and is currently in use in over 5,000 schools across the country. Recently, the Check-In, Check-Out (CICO) component of the SWIS was added to allow schools to easily summarize DPR data. There are some costs associated with using both the SWIS and the SWIS-CICO. Additional information regarding these programs can be found at *www.swis.org*. The SWIS-CICO allows schools to track not only percentage of points for the whole school day but also the percentage of points earned each class period. In addition, the SWIS-CICO allows school staff to simultaneously view ODR data and DPR data. Figure 7.1 provides an SWIS-CICO summary of an individual student's DPR data over a 1-month period. The SWIS-CICO allows schools to set each student's goal. In Figure 7.1 the goal is set at 80% of points. The SWIS-CICO also allows schools to document absences, missing data, and if the BEP has been modified (as indicated by a vertical line on the graph). Figure 7.1 illustrates the data from a single class period for one student, as summarized by the SWIS-CICO. The multiple-period report illustrated in Figure 7.2 alerts the behavior support team to the fact that the student is consistently falling far below his percentage point goal during third period. Based on this data, the team would probably conclude additional assessment and possible modifications may be needed for the student during that period.

For schools that are not using the SWIS-CICO, the Microsoft Excel graphing program is available on Leanne Hawken's website (*www.ed.utah.edu/~hawken_l/bep.htm*). This program allows schools to enter the percentage of points and the data will be automatically graphed. The

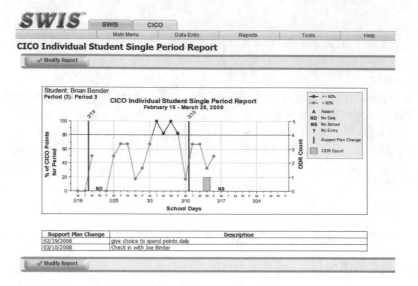

FIGURE 7.1. Individual student graph from the SWIS-CICO for one class period. Reprinted with permission from *www.SWIS-CICO* v0.9 May & Talmadge.

program will also allow schools to change each student's goal if individualization of daily point goals is necessary.

Other Data to Document Response to the BEP Intervention

Additional data should be collected to assess overall student response to the BEP. These data include the number of (1) ODRs, (2) absences and/or tardies, (3) students needing Tier III support, and (4) referrals to special education for behavior problems. Data on academic measures should also be gathered to determine if there is an increase in performance.

Students are typically referred to the BEP after receiving a criterion number of ODRs. Examining if there is a reduction in ODRs following BEP implementation will provide an addi-

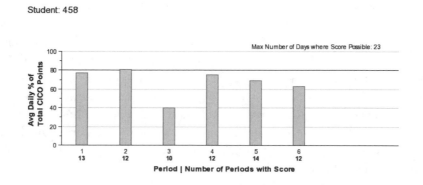

FIGURE 7.2. SWIS-CICO report across class periods for an individual student. Reprinted with permission from *www.SWIS-CICO* v0.9 May & Talmadge.

tional measure of how the student is doing. Schools that are implementing the BEP should have a standardized method of collecting and organizing ODRs. Data collection is typically established as part of the Tier I/Tier II-level prevention program. It should be noted that some students will not show dramatic reductions in ODRs following BEP implementation, but rather will show a "leveling off" trend in their data. This indicates that the BEP is helping to prevent further escalation.

Many students who can benefit from the BEP have excessive numbers of absences and tardies. These data should also be examined pre- and postimplementation. Although the BEP does not target absences and tardies directly, we have noticed students' attendance typically improves with placement on the BEP. We hypothesize that this correlation is due to the increased accountability created by daily contact with a caring adult.

One goal of the BEP is to teach students prosocial skills, to prevent them from needing more intensive and costly behavior supports, such as special education. Schools should track the number of students who require Tier III support prior to and following BEP implementation. In addition, to underscore the preventative impact of the BEP, schools should track the number of students who are referred for special education services for behavior problems (i.e., for an emotional and behavior disability) pre- and post-BEP implementation. Previous research has found that effective implementation of the BEP led to a reduction in students needing Tier III levels of support and special education (Hawken et al., 2007). This type of data should be shared with school and district-level personnel to highlight the cost savings associated with implementing the BEP.

The BEP has been shown to increase academic engagement and decrease problem behavior (Hawken & Horner, 2003). It is hypothesized that increased academic engagement, coupled with effective instruction, will lead to increases in academic performance. Many of the modifications to the high school BEP (described in detail in Chapter 9) involve improving skills that should lead to increases in academic performance, for example, study skills and organizational skills. Therefore, we assume that participating in the BEP will result in increased academic achievement. More research is needed on the connection between implementation of the BEP and improved academic performance but schools can keep track of data such as the percent of work completion, grades, scores on curriculum-based measures, and scores on end-of-the-year high-stakes tests to document BEP effects on academic achievement.

BEP Acceptability Data

It is important to get feedback from staff, parents, and students to determine how "consumers" of the BEP feel about the intervention. If teachers who are implementing the BEP do not feel that it is effective or worth their time and effort, they will be much less likely to implement the intervention. Overall, we have found that the BEP receives high acceptability ratings across teachers, parents, and students. Examples of BEP acceptability questionnaires for teachers, students, and parents are included in Appendices F.2, F.3, and F.4. These questionnaires address how staff and parents feel about whether or not the BEP worked for an individual student. They also provide the student with an opportunity to voice his or her opinion on how the intervention is working. We also recommend that the entire school staff be surveyed to determine if any programmatic modifications to the BEP intervention are needed within a particular school.

FADING STUDENTS FROM THE BEP INTERVENTION

The BEP team may be tempted to leave a student on the BEP indefinitely, even after a student has demonstrated consistent, significant improvement in behavior. The team may worry that the student's behavior will regress if he or she does not receive the continued support of the BEP. Keeping each student on the BEP until the end of the academic year becomes the default option for many schools. This approach, however, can unnecessarily overburden the BEP team.

For middle and high schools, we recommend that the BEP roster consist of no more than 30 students per BEP coordinator. Beyond 30 students, it becomes difficult to effectively manage the program and respond to issues that arise. For elementary school, we recommend a maximum of 15–20 students per BEP coordinator. Elementary school students often need more prompting, or the coordinator needs to check in and check out with the students in their classrooms. It is more time-intensive for the elementary school BEP coordinator to manage the intervention than it is at the middle or high school level. Fading students from the BEP intervention once their behavior improvements are sustainable increases the efficiency of the BEP and is a wise use of resources. At the same time, the team must avoid removing a student whose behavior would deteriorate without the support that the BEP provides.

Determining the Appropriate Time to Fade a Student from the BEP

The team should begin by looking at the BEP data. We recommend that the BEP team consider fading on at least a quarterly basis, preferably more often if the number of students on the BEP is exceeding its capacity. If this is a regularly occurring agenda item, there will be fewer tendencies to maintain students on an intervention that they no longer need. For many schools, the timing of considering the need to fade students coincides with grading or marking periods.

The BEP coordinator will bring the BEP graphs, as usual, to the behavior support team meeting. These graphs can be printed to show a student's data over a few days or several weeks. For a decision regarding fading, graphs should illustrate long-term data. Prior to the meeting, the coordinator can go through the graphs and identify students who have consistently met their BEP percentage point goals for at least 4 weeks. These students have demonstrated a consistent pattern of desired behavior and may be ready to maintain their behavior without the support of the BEP.

The BEP coordinator can circle the graphs of each of these students, and provide copies for each behavior support team member. Figure 7.3 provides an example of DPR data that might indicate that a student is ready to be removed from the BEP. In this example, Milo has had a few days below his 80% point goal, but overall he is consistently meeting and exceeding this goal, with many 100% days.

Each behavior support team should develop its own criteria for fading. In some schools, an average performance of 80% or more points across 4 weeks indicates a student may be ready to fade off the intervention. Other schools have chosen a 6-week criterion. A key point when developing a criterion for fading is that it should be based on an average or on a majority of days rather than on consecutive performance. For example, a student should receive above 80% of points the majority of the time (or on average) versus the student must *always* receive above 80% and one tough day of 70% disqualifies him or her for the fading discussion The latter criterion may be too stringent.

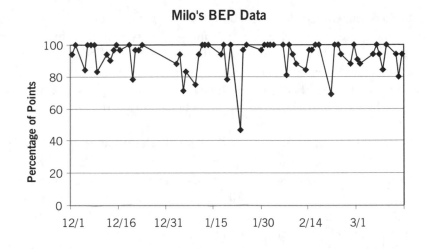

FIGURE 7.3. Student BEP graph indicating that fading may be appropriate.

As a behavior support team, the group should discuss each possible fading candidate. The team can raise any concerns they may have about removing an individual from the BEP. A team member may have information about a student that persuades the team that the student will be unable to maintain behavioral gains without the BEP. Alternatively, the BEP may be written into a student's IEP behavioral goals. In this case, the student cannot be removed from the BEP intervention unless an IEP meeting is convened and the IEP team agrees that the BEP should be removed and the IEP should be changed. If the team decides to remove a student from the BEP, they should initiate a gradual fading process rather than an immediate termination of the program for the student. For maximum effectiveness, we recommend incorporating a self-management component to scaffold the student's appropriate behavior as BEP support is faded.

Using Self-Management to Fade BEP Support

The goal of self-management is to increase the student's sense of responsibility and ability to manage his or her own behavior without the need for redirection, prompting, and management by an adult figure. Self-management should be introduced before BEP support is faded.

We suggest that the self-management component look similar to the DPR. The goal is to shift from teacher ratings of the student's behavior to student ratings of his or her own behavior. Initially, the student and the teacher will rate the student's behavior simultaneously. Both individuals will have his or her own copy of the DPR. At the end of the class period, the teacher and student should compare behavior ratings. At this point, the student is learning to rate his or her own behavior. Success is defined as a *match between the student's score and the teacher's score* (even if both individuals rate a behavior as a "0"). If there is a discrepancy between the two scores, the teacher and student should discuss the discrepancy and the reason for the teacher's decision. The teacher's score is assumed to be the accurate score. The emphasis of this first stage is for the student's ratings to come closer and closer to consistently approximating the teacher's ratings, until the student is reliably and accurately rating his or her own behavior.

In order to encourage the student's reliability in scoring, the student can earn small rewards for having the same score as the teacher. For example, if a student gives him- or herself a rating of 1, 1, 1, 2 on the four behavior goals, and the teacher gives the same rating, the student could earn a schoolwide token or bonus points on the DPR. Typically, this would be discouraged because the student should not earn additional reinforcement for suboptimal behavior. In the early stages of BEP removal, however, the student earns rewards for accuracy and honesty rather than for behavior.

Once the student can consistently rate his or her behavior reliably (i.e., 80–85% agreement between teacher and student), rewards for accuracy can be faded, and rewards for appropriate behavior can be reinstated. The next goal is to remove the teacher rating component. The number of times that the teacher provides a rating is gradually reduced. For example, during the first week of BEP removal, the teacher will provide a rating on 4 of 5 days. The student rating is used once. In the next week, the teacher provides ratings on 3 days.

In addition to fading teacher ratings, the student's participation in the check-in/check-out process can be faded as well. While the student is learning to self-assess his or her behavior, he or she continues to check in and check out and to turn in a DPR. The BEP coordinator continues to collect, enter, and analyze the student's BEP data during the time that he or she is learning to rate his or her own behavior. Data collection at this point is critical. The BEP data will demonstrate whether the student's behavior stays the same, improves, or significantly worsens, as the BEP is gradually faded. In the case of worsening behavior, the team should discuss whether or not the student is ready to move to self-management. The worsening behavior may be an indication that it is too early to remove the BEP support. Alternatively, it may be an indication that the BEP fading process has not been adequately explained to the student, or effectively implemented.

A clear conversation between the student and an adult regarding the goals and process of the self-management strategy is critical to its success. Any member of the BEP team may lead this discussion with the student. We recommend using someone who knows the student well and whom the student views as actively involved in the BEP process. During this discussion, the adult should explain to the student that he or she is pleased with the student's behavioral improvements and believes the student has demonstrated maturity and a readiness to be responsible for his or her own behavior. The adult should share a copy of the student's data with him or her. These data should already be familiar to the student, but the emphasis in this conversation is to demonstrate the student's consistent performance above the 80% goal. The adult should then explain that the student's accomplishment will be recognized by allowing the student to become a self-manager, without need for the BEP. Finally, the adult should explain what the student can expect as the BEP system is gradually faded. The adult should have the student practice using the self-management DPR several times. The student should leave this meeting feeling a sense of pride and accomplishment in his or her behavioral accomplishments as well as motivation to continue to demonstrate appropriate behavior.

Increasing Success in Fading BEP Support

To increase chances of a successful fading process, it will be important to talk with the parents and students about fading when initial BEP training takes place. That is, when the student learns about the intervention and how to participate, fading should be discussed with a brief mention of how, and potentially when, fading will occur. We have noticed that when students and parents know the goal of the BEP is for students to eventually graduate and self-monitor their own behavior, there is less surprise and more acceptance when the time comes for fading the student off the intervention.

An additional way to increase the success of fading the BEP intervention is to transfer the adult attention component to another adult in the school building. One important reason why students do not want to be removed from the BEP intervention is that they enjoy the extra adult attention and reinforcement. This is particularly true for elementary age students. We have found it helpful to plan for other opportunities and experiences that will allow the student to gain access to adult attention. For example, the student can serve in an alumni role and assist the BEP coordinator in checking students in and out. He or she could also help with setting up and organizing reinforcers, making copies of lottery tickets, or other tasks related to implementing the BEP. He or she could become an assistant to another adult in the school building, for example, the librarian or the computer lab teacher. Providing students with leadership roles will increase their chances of successfully fading from the BEP intervention and becoming more involved in roles that are naturally occurring in the school system.

Graduation and Alumni Parties

Another strategy for increasing the success of the fading process is to hold a BEP graduation celebration once the student has completely and successfully been removed from the BEP. Some schools have scheduled a 30-minute party during lunch time that both the student and his or her parent can attend to celebrate successful graduation from the BEP intervention. We encourage schools to invite the classroom teacher or teachers if possible to also join in on the celebration as they are an integral part of successful BEP implementation. Figure 7.4 provides a sample diploma from Vista Elementary School. The diploma is signed by the school psychologist, social worker, and the principal. Other schools may choose to have the classroom teacher or teachers also sign the diploma.

Students should be provided incentives for managing their own behavior and for continuing to be successful without the support of the BEP intervention. Some schools implement a quarterly "BEP alumni" party for students who have graduated from the BEP and have not received any ODRs for problem behavior during the quarter. Alumni parties have included activities such as pizza during lunch time (often donated by a community restaurant), root beer float parties during the last 30 minutes of school, or 30 minutes of game time with snacks during which each BEP alumni can bring a friend.

Weekly BEP alumni check-outs are another way to additionally reinforce students for appropriate behavior. One school instituted a weekly check-out for BEP alumni during which students could receive a small reinforcer (e.g., snack) for continuing to be successful without the BEP intervention. For many of our schools, managing the check-out process with BEP alumni along with current BEP students is too much to do on a weekly basis, but if your school has a limited number of students on the BEP this may be an option.

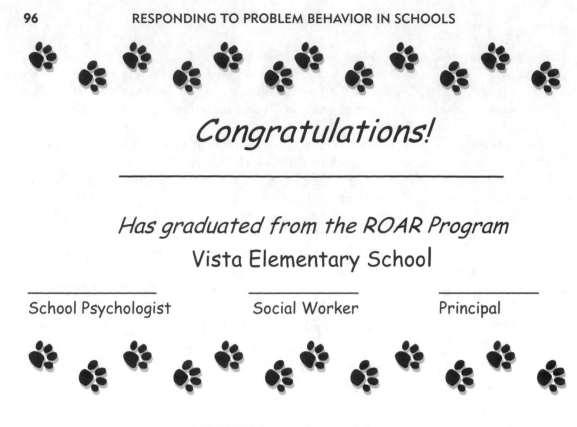

FIGURE 7.4. Sample BEP diploma.

What If the Student Wants to Stay on the BEP Intervention?

We have found that, in schools where the BEP intervention is running well, students like being on the BEP. Students view the program positively. A student may view BEP removal as a punishment rather than as a recognition or promotion. The student may, in fact, respond by increasing his or her inappropriate behavior. This is why it is important to talk about fading during the initial training on the BEP. In addition, as mentioned previously, we have found that providing students with alternative ways to gain adult attention such as becoming the BEP coordinator's helper allows students to continue to feel supported without needing full access to the intervention.

If a middle school or high school student wants to stay on the BEP, he or she could continue to check in and check out with the BEP coordinator (unless, of course, the additional check-in/check-out overburdens the coordinator). At the middle school or high school level, this should not pose an unnecessary burden on the resources of the behavior support team. The student continues to rate him- or herself on the DPR, rather than taking the teacher's time. Although the student may elect to continue to check in and check out, the behavior support team no longer enters, analyzes, or responds to the data. They simply file the student's DPR in the student's folder. The student can continue to have daily contact with a person he or she enjoys without creating any additional workload for the behavior support team. This makes it possible for a new student to begin the BEP in his or her place.

Final Consideration for Fading

One final consideration in terms of fading students from the BEP intervention is timing in relation to the end of the school year. Often, the easiest transition is to discontinue the BEP intervention at the end of the school year. Rather than implementing the self-management process, we have found that treating the end of the school year as a natural fade has worked with many students. A celebration is provided at the end of the school year and students are told that they will begin the next school year as BEP alumni. This type of natural fading works well with the majority of students who have demonstrated success on the BEP. Some students do continue to need BEP support the following school year. This end-of-year option is workable only if your BEP intervention has not reached the maximum number of students it can support. If there are already 30 students on the intervention, and three additional students need to be added, the fading procedures described above should be implemented so that the BEP coordinator is not overwhelmed with too many students at one time.

CHAPTER 8

The Modified BEP
Adaptations and Elaborations

The BEP is efficient because it uses a common organizing structure to respond to a group of students with similar behavioral needs. Applying the same intervention for 30 students is far cheaper and swifter than creating 30 individualized responses. The efficacy of a common approach does, however, have limitations. The BEP may be an inadequate response to the behavioral needs of some students for a variety of reasons:

1. The BEP is contraindicated given the function of the student's problem behavior.
2. The BEP provides only one part of the full spectrum of support required by the student.
3. The student is not an appropriate candidate for the BEP.

In this chapter we discuss BEP modifications and elaborations that address the first two issues. Identification of appropriate candidates for the BEP was discussed in Chapter 3.

WHEN DOES IT MAKE SENSE TO USE A MODIFIED BEP?

The BEP team briefly screens all BEP referrals to decide whether a student is an appropriate candidate for the program. Once a student passes this simple screen, the student begins the basic BEP. Daily behavioral data is immediately available for each student on the BEP. The behavior support team should consider a modified BEP if the basic BEP is ineffective. We suggest that the student participate and that the team collects BEP data for at least 2–3 weeks before considering a modified BEP.

Is the BEP effective for this student? The behavior support team can answer this question if (1) the student has a specific, measurable, behavior goal; and (2) BEP data have been collected and recorded, consistently and accurately. Both criteria are easily met when the BEP system is implemented with fidelity.

For most BEP students, the measurable goal will be "Student will earn at least 80% of possible points each day." For students who are initially incapable of succeeding at this level, the behavior support team may adjust this goal downward.

To determine if the BEP is working for a specific student, the behavior support team examines the student's data graphs. *Is the student meeting his or her BEP goal on at least 4 out of 5 days? If the student is not meeting that goal, how discrepant is the student's performance?* The team is less likely to be concerned about a student who consistently earns 70% of points than a student who earns less than 50% of points on a daily basis. Another way to determine whether the student is making progress is to compare baseline percentage of points earned with points earned following BEP implementation. In addition to percentage of points earned, the team can look for other important patterns. *Does the student frequently forget to pick up the DPR in the morning or refuse to turn it in at the end of the day? Does the student consistently meet his or her goal on Tuesday, Wednesday, and Thursday, but have significant behavioral problems on Monday and Friday? What other data patterns does the team observe?* If schools are using the SWIS-CICO data system, the behavior support teams can also examine data by time of day.

If the team determines that the program is ineffective for a specific student, they should brainstorm strategies for modifying the basic BEP in a manner that will improve its effectiveness for that student. Team members should consider the simplest solutions first. For example, a student who is not picking up the DPR in the morning may have a difficult relationship with the person who runs morning check-in, and may be trying to avoid that person. The team may consider identifying an adult who has a special connection with the student. The student could check in with the other adult instead.

A student who consistently refuses to return the DPR with a parent signature may be getting in serious trouble at home for less-than-perfect performance. The BEP coordinator may review the home component guidelines with the parent, or the team may decide to eliminate the parent signature requirement for this student. In such a case, some schools have assigned the student to a "surrogate parent," such as a teacher, educational assistant, or janitor in the school. The surrogate parent signs the form and provides the student with additional positive feedback on his or her behavior.

In some cases, the level of support provided is not adequate to meet the student's behavioral needs. For example, a student may be consistently participating in the BEP but continues to earn only 50% of his or her points on a daily basis. The student may require additional supports, such as academic interventions or an individualized behavior support plan (BSP).

USING FUNCTIONAL BEHAVIORAL ASSESSMENT TO MODIFY THE BEP

One of the early steps in creating a modified BEP is to conduct a brief functional behavioral assessment (FBA). The FBA is a method of gathering information about the events that predict and maintain problem behavior (Crone & Horner, 2003). This information can be used to determine the reason that a student acts in a certain way under certain conditions. The FBA helps identify the *function* of the problem behavior.

Students' problem behavior can be broadly grouped into two categories: (1) problem behavior that is maintained by obtaining access to desirable stimuli (e.g., attention, activities, objects) and (2) problem behavior that is maintained by escaping or avoiding undesirable stimuli (e.g., activities, events, demands). FBAs can be fairly simple and brief, or complex and time-consuming. The complexity of the assessment will depend on the complexity and severity of the problem behavior. When used in conjunction with the BEP, we suggest conducting a simple FBA to identify the conditions most likely to result in problem behavior, and the consequences most likely to maintain the problem behavior for the identified student. A student whose behavior is complex or severe and who requires a full FBA (for the difference between a full FBA and a simple FBA, refer to Crone & Horner, 2003) will not be an appropriate candidate for the BEP. A simple FBA consists of interviewing one or more teachers. Typically, the referring teacher is the one interviewed. Often, older students (e.g., in upper elementary, middle, or high school) can provide information related to why they are engaging in problem behavior so in these cases a brief student interview is also recommended.

Behavior Maintained by the Desire to Obtain Something

Students in this category engage in problem behavior because it results in obtaining something that they want. Students may want to obtain a toy, time to play on the playground, or attention from their peers or adults. The desire to obtain attention is a common function of misbehavior. Attention can be either positive or negative. For example, a teacher might reprimand the student in front of the class (negative attention) or a peer might laugh along with an inappropriate joke (positive attention). Some problem behaviors of these students might include talking back to the teacher, arguing or fighting with students, refusing to work, or disrupting the class.

Escape-Maintained Behavior

The problem behaviors exhibited by students in this category are often indistinguishable from problem behaviors that are maintained by the desire to obtain attention or other stimuli. The difference between the two groups is the function that the behavior serves for the student. Students in this group may be disruptive, talk back to the teacher, and argue with their peers in order to get out of a situation or to get away from a person. For example, a student who dislikes male teachers may throw frequent tantrums in male-led classes if she has discovered that tantrums in class get her sent to the office (and away from the male teacher). A student who has difficulty interacting with peers may be disruptive during lunch so that he is sent to the principal's office. By engaging in disruptive behavior, the student has been removed from (i.e., escaped) an unpleasant social situation. Students may also engage in disruptive behavior in order to escape a task that it too difficult, long, or boring for them.

Academic-Related Problem Behavior

Students with behavioral problems often have problems organizing and completing academic work. The problem behavior of students in this group is related directly to the responsibilities of completing academic tasks consistently, accurately, and on time. Students in this category typically have trouble with the following types of tasks: (1) bringing the necessary materials to class, (2) arriving at class on time, (3) completing assignments on time, (4) turning in assignments, (5) being neat and organized, and (6) following directions. For these students, problem behaviors arise because of poor attention, poor organization, or poor memory rather than defiance, aggression, or poor social skills. An FBA may demonstrate that the student would benefit from academic assessment and academic support in addition to the BEP.

MODIFYING THE BEP
TO FIT THE NEEDS OF A WIDER VARIETY OF STUDENTS

The basic BEP works most effectively for students with attention-motivated problem behavior and/or for students who find adult attention reinforcing (Hawken & Horner, 2003; March & Horner, 2002). The system is structured so that students receive a positive adult contact at least twice a day. Furthermore, students receive feedback on their behavior throughout the day. On a nightly basis, students receive parental attention for their school behavior. To the extent that teachers and parents attend to and encourage students' appropriate behavior, this behavior will improve. Slight modifications to the content or process of the basic BEP can improve their usefulness for students with academic-related problem behavior or escape-motivated problem behavior, as well as for students with attention-motivated behavior.

Modifying the BEP for Adult Attention-Motivated Behavior

The basic BEP may be inadequate for some students with attention-motivated behavior. Although the basic BEP addresses the appropriate function of the problem behavior, the intervention may not be strong enough to create change in the student's behavior. The team may need to elaborate on the basic BEP in order to help the student meet his or her behavioral goal. For example, the team may decide that this student needs more frequent feedback and attention than the basic BEP provides. The team may modify the BEP to allow for more frequent interactions between the student and instructors. For example, some schools that we have worked with have implemented a midday check-in with the BEP coordinator for students who need additional attention. Alternatively, the team may suggest adding a self-monitoring and self-reinforcement package to the BEP for a student. As a third possibility, the team may suggest adding more powerful reinforcers for the student. For example, the student may respond more favorably to attention from a particular individual. Perhaps the student has a special connection with the librarian or the school custodian. One modification that the team could build in is the opportunity to either receive feedback from this individual or to spend an extra 5–10 minutes with this person if the student meets his or her 80% goal for that day. Figure 8.1 provides an example of a completed contract for a modified BEP for a student with attention-motivated behavior (see Appendix G.1 for a blank contract).

Modifying the BEP for Peer Attention-Motivated Behavior

Many students, particularly older students, engage in problem behavior to get attention from their peers/friends. For example, a student may talk out in class or make sarcastic comments to the teacher to get friends to laugh with him or her. As students get older, peer attention tends to be more reinforcing than adult attention. Possible BEP modifications for students who have peer attention-motivated problem behavior include having the student earn reinforcers to share

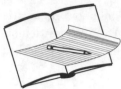

I, _Jasmine Jackson_____, agree to work on these things this year.

1. _Be respectful toward teachers_____

2. _Play safely on the playground_____

3. _Keep my hands and feet to self_____

I will work with _Mrs. Jennings (music teacher)_____ to keep track of my progress.
I understand that I will have a chance to earn a reward each week when I meet my goals. A list of
rewards I would like to earn include:

1. _10 minutes with Mrs. Jennings to learn to play guitar_____

2. _Extra time in music class with Mrs. Jennings_____

3. _Time to help Mrs. Jennings put musical instruments away_____

I will try hard to do my best to meet these goals every day.

_Jasmine Jackson_____
Signature of Student

I will do my best to help _Jasmine_____ meet his/her goals every day.

_Mrs. Jennings_____   _Mr. Jackson_____
Signature of Coordinator   Signature of Parent

FIGURE 8.1. Example of a completed contract for a modified BEP for a student with attention-motivated behavior.

with peers such as coupons to the snack bar or snacks after school. One of the main reinforcers used to effectively engage these students are activity-based reinforcers. For example, students can earn extra gym time or computer time and can invite five friends to participate in the activity. For elementary school students, BEP students can earn extra recess for the class by meeting their daily point goals after a prespecified number of days. It is often effective (and efficient) to ask students directly what types of activities they would like to earn for reinforcers that can be shared with friends.

Modifying the BEP for Escape-Motivated Behavior

Responding effectively to this type of problem behavior within the BEP intervention requires creativity. If a student's problem behavior is motivated by the desire to escape authority figures, the student will not respond well to an intervention that significantly increases the number of adult contacts throughout the day. In fact, this type of system could worsen the student's problem behavior (March & Horner, 2002). We suggest the following possible modifications:

1. Do not require the student to check in/check out directly with the BEP coordinator. Rather, the student can pick up a DPR from a designated box and return it to the box at the end of the day. The student is still responsible for giving the DPR to his or her teachers throughout the day.
2. The points earned on the DPR can be used to "purchase" personally meaningful reinforcers. For example, a student who has escape-motivated behavior might want to earn 10 minutes of time listening to music as a way to escape a class that he dislikes. Another student may wish to earn reading time during a homeroom period she finds particularly boring.
3. Even if a student generally avoids adult interaction, there may be one adult with whom he or she has a close connection. This individual may be utilized as the point of contact for check-in and check-out.
4. For some students, the function of the problem behavior may be to escape a task that is academically difficult for them. In this case, the student may respond to the attention aspect of the BEP, but may require academic intervention as well.

Figure 8.2 provides an example of a list of modifications for a BEP for a student with escape-motivated behavior.

Modified BEP

Attention Teachers:

Randall Prima will be placed on a modified BEP. The following modifications will be made.

1. Rate Randall's behavior on his DPR each class period. However, rather than discussing it with him, write your comments on the card and hand it back to him.
2. Randall will discuss his daily performance, and opportunities for improvement, with Mr. Reynolds, his football coach.
3. When Randall meets his goal for the week, he can choose from a range of personally meaningful reinforcers. Mr. Reynolds will coordinate the receipt of reinforcers.

Randall's reinforcers are listed below:

1. Time to work as office aide rather than attend homeroom.
2. Early dismissal from class one period per day.
3. 10-minutes time in gym with a friend after classwork is completed, once per day.
4. Time to be a peer mentor in younger grade classrooms, once per week.

If you have any questions, please contact Chris Grayson, the BEP coordinator.

Thank you.

FIGURE 8.2. List of modifications for BEP for a student with escape-motivated behavior.

BEP Plus Academic Supports

A student who has significant difficulty with organization, task completion, and ability to focus may benefit from modified BEP *goals*. Goals listed on the basic BEP are typically behavioral in nature and broad in scope (e.g., Be respectful, Be safe). Goals listed on a modified BEP can be academic in nature, and more specific. The modified BEP could include the following type of goals:

1. Begin work immediately.
2. Complete assignment.
3. Turn assignment in on time.
4. Arrive at class on time.
5. Arrive at class with all necessary materials and books.

In this case, the modified BEP acts as a constant reminder to the student about what he or she needs to do to succeed academically. This is helpful because many of these students have difficulty with memory, attention, and organization. Figure 8.3 provides an example of a modified BEP with academic goals.

The student may require academic support in addition to modified BEP goals. In this case, the behavior support team may recommend that (1) an academic assessment to determine the student's skill and performance deficits, and (2) the student receive academic interventions such as tutoring or after-school support to remediate academic deficits.

Daily Progress Report

Name: _____   Points received: _____

Date: _____   Points possible: _____

Daily goal reached?   **YES   NO**

0 = No   1 = So-so   2 = Yes

Goal	A.M.	P.E./Music	Reading	Math	P.M.
Begin work immediately.					
Complete assignment.					
Turn assignment in on time.					
Arrive to class on time.					
Arrive to class with all necessary materials and books.					

Teacher comments: _____

Parent comments: _____

Parent signature: _____

FIGURE 8.3. Modified BEP with academic goals.

FUNCTIONAL BEHAVIORAL ASSESSMENT

The modified BEP should have the greatest positive impact when the modifications are matched directly to the needs of the student. A mismatch between student and the modified BEP can, at the least, have no impact on the student's behavior, and, at the worst, cause the student's behavior to deteriorate. Due to constraints on time and resources, most schools need to produce the greatest impact on student behavior in the most efficient manner. Appropriate BEP modifications can be identified through effective assessment. *It is critical, however, that the assessment is brief and simple.* A complicated or time-consuming assessment procedure would eliminate the BEP's primary advantage, that is, efficiency of response. We suggest using FBA to identify appropriate BEP modifications for a particular student.

There are a wide variety of methods to conduct an FBA, ranging from a brief, semistructured interview to a comprehensive interview coupled with observations in the classroom. To obtain the necessary information for the modified BEP, a brief or "simple" FBA is the most appropriate place to begin.

Simple FBA

The simple FBA is a brief, structured interview. The interview is conducted with the teacher(s) or staff member(s) who referred the student to the behavior support team. The interview can be conducted by a behavior support team member, school psychologist, behavior support specialist, or other person with adequate training and skill. The desired outcomes of the FBA are to (1) obtain an observable and measurable description of the problem behavior, (2) identify the setting events or antecedents that predict when the behavior will and will not occur, and (3) identify the consequences that maintain the problem behavior (O'Neill et al., 1997). This information can be used to determine if the student's problem behavior is escape-motivated, attention-motivated, or primarily a result of an academic or organizational deficit.

There are several FBA interview instruments in print. Two similar instruments, the teacher interview of the Functional Behavioral Assessment—Behavior Support Plan Protocol (F-BSP Protocol) and the Functional Assessment Checklist for Teachers (FACTS) will be presented here. Each school may choose to use a different FBA interview. An adequate interview includes the following critical features:

1. It can be completed in 20 minutes or less.
2. It identifies the specific problem behavior.
3. It identifies the routines that support problem behavior.
4. It identifies the "function" of the problem behavior. Each of the interview instruments discussed in this chapter meet all four criteria.

Case Example

The following case example demonstrates how to use the simple FBA to determine the type of BEP modifications that may be most appropriate for an individual student. In each example interview, the student and problem (i.e., incomplete assignments) remain the same, but the reason (function) for the problem behavior changes.

Background Information

Randall is a sixth-grade student at Fairview Middle School. He is well liked by the other students. He has a good sense of humor and is on several athletic teams, including soccer and football. Randall is struggling academically. On his most recent report card, he received a D in math and failing grades in social studies and English. His poor grades in each of these classes are due primarily to a significant number of incomplete or missing class assignments. During the same grading period, Randall also received an A in physical education and a B in industrial arts. Randall is referred to the behavior support team by his social studies/English teacher, Mrs. Nielsen.

BEP Plus Academic Supports

Mr. Jensen, the school counselor and a member of the behavior support team, interviews Mrs. Nielsen. In this interview the description of the problem behavior is the most revealing. As Mrs. Nielsen describes Randall's poor work completion, it becomes clear that he has trouble remembering to bring assignments and materials to class, is unorganized, and has trouble paying attention in class. He does not appear to be gaining anything specific from this behavior. For example, he sits quietly at his desk, not talking with or receiving attention from his peers. He is not escaping work or the situation, as he is never sent out of the classroom and Mrs. Nielsen requires him to continue to work throughout the class period. In this example, it appears that Randall would benefit from a BEP with academic supports. The team could recommend at least three options:

1. Modify the goals of the BEP to reflect specific, organizational goals.
2. Conduct an academic assessment to determine the student's academic performance level.
3. Modify the student's curriculum and assignment to more closely reflect his or her skill level.

The results of this interview using the F-BSP Protocol are illustrated in Figure 8.4.

BEP Plus Modifications for Attention-Motivated Behavior

Now, examine the interview presented in Figure 8.5. In this case, we demonstrate the same interview format and teacher, but with a different set of responses. In this example, Mrs. Nielsen indicates that Randall frequently becomes teary-eyed and withdrawn when he is given a lengthy written assignment in class. This behavior results in concern from his teacher and friends, who try to cheer him up. In the end, his assignments remain undone or incomplete. Information gathered from Randall's math and social studies teachers confirms a similar pattern of behavior. Academic assessments indicate that Randall is capable of completing the assignments at the level they are currently provided.

This example illustrates the same student with the same concern, but in this case, it is clear that the problem behavior is not due to lack of organization and performance skills. Rather, the

(text continues on page 111)

FUNCTIONAL BEHAVIORAL ASSESSMENT INTERVIEW—TEACHER/STAFF/PARENT

Student name: _Randall_   Age: _13_   Grade: _6_   Date: _12/2/09_

Person(s) interviewed: _Mrs. Nielsen_

Interviewer: _Mr. Jensen_

Student Profile: What is the student good at or what are some strengths that the student brings to school?

Has a good sense of humor, is athletic, and is well liked by other students.

Step 1: Interview Teacher/Staff/Parent
Description of the Behavior

> **What does the problem behavior(s) look like?**
> Incomplete and missing assignments; Randall forgets to bring his materials (e.g., binder, pencil, paper) to class and often forgets his homework.
>
> **How often does the problem behavior(s) occur?**
> Assignments are missing on a weekly basis in Math, Social Studies, and English
>
> **How long does the problem behavior(s) last when it does occur?**
> If Randall forgets his materials and homework, it can disrupt the whole period because he is not ready to go over the homework and is unprepared for new lesson.
>
> **How disruptive or dangerous is the problem behavior(s)?**
> Behavior is not dangerous but is disruptive to his academic performance. At risk for being retained.

Description of the Antecedents
Identifying Routines: When, where, and with whom are problem behaviors most likely?

Schedule (Times)	Activity	Specific Problem Behavior	Likelihood of Problem Behavior	With Whom Does Problem Occur?
8:30–9:30	Math	Unorganized/forgets homework	Low High 1 2 3 4 (5) 6	Mrs. Singh
9:30–10:30	Physical Education		(1) 2 3 4 5 6	Mr. Woods
10:30–11:30	Social Studies	Unorganized/forgets homework	1 2 3 4 5 (6)	Mrs. Nielsen
11:30–12:00	Lunch		(1) 2 3 4 5 6	
12:00–12:30	Homeroom		(1) 2 3 4 5 6	Mr. Sanchez
12:30–1:30	English/Language Arts	Unorganized/forgets homework	1 2 3 4 5 (6)	Mrs. Nielsen
1:30–2:30	Science	Unorganized/forgets homework	1 2 3 (4) 5 6	Mrs. Avila
2:30–3:30	Industrial Arts		(1) 2 3 4 5 6	Mr. Carpenter

(cont.)

FIGURE 8.4. Example of a completed F-BSP teacher interview demonstrating a need for BEP plus academic supports.

Summarize Antecedents (and Setting Events)

> **What situations seem to set off the problem behavior?** (difficult tasks, transitions, structured activities, small-group settings, teacher's request, particular individuals, etc.)
> Classes that require homework and organization with materials.
>
> **When is the problem behavior most likely to occur?** (times of day and days of the week)
> During Social Studies, English, and Math. It also happens in Science but not as often due to the "hands on" nature of the class (not as much homework).
>
> **When is the problem behavior least likely to occur?** (times of day and days of the week)
> During P.E., Industrial Arts, Lunch and Homeroom.
>
> **Setting Events: Are there specific conditions, events, or activities that make the problem behavior worse?** (missed medication, history of academic failure, conflict at home, missed meals, lack of sleep, history of problems with peers, etc.)
> None identified.

Description of the Consequences

> **What ususally happens after the behavior occurs?** (what is the teacher's reaction, how do other students react, is the student sent to the office, does the student get out of doing work, does the student get in a power struggle, etc.)
> He receives reprimands from his teachers and parents, and ultimately receives poor grades. He's required to continue to do his work in class—does not get sent out of class.

- - - - - - End of Interview - - - - - -

Step 2: Propose a Testable Explanation

Setting Events	Antecedents	Behaviors	Consequences
	Classes requiring organization/homework (e.g., Math, Social Studies)	1. Doesn't complete homework 2. Comes to class without materials	Poor grades

Function of the Behavior

For each ABC sequence listed above, why do you think the behavior is occurring? (to get teacher attention, peer attention, desired object/activity, or escape undesirable activity, demand particular people, etc.)

1. When taking a class that requires homework, organization, and materials, Randall appears to have difficulty remembering homework assignments and organizing materials, which results in poor grades in those classes.

How confident are you that your testable explanation is accurate?

Very sure			So-so			Not at all sure
6	⑤	4	3	2		1

FIGURE 8.4. *(cont.)*

FUNCTIONAL BEHAVIORAL ASSESSMENT INTERVIEW—TEACHER/STAFF/PARENT

Student name: Randall   Age: 13   Grade: 6   Date: 12/2/09

Person(s) interviewed: Mrs. Nielsen

Interviewer: Mr. Jensen

Student Profile: What is the student good at or what are some strengths that the student brings to school?

Has a good sense of humor, is athletic, and is well liked by other students.

Step 1: Interview Teacher/Staff/Parent
Description of the Behavior

> **What does the problem behavior(s) look like?**
> Randall becomes teary-eyed and refuses to do work (sits with arms crossed, head down) when given a written assignment.
>
> **How often does the problem behavior(s) occur?**
> Four to five times a week when written assignments are given.
>
> **How long does the problem behavior(s) last when it does occur?**
> Randall cries and refuses to do work until friends and teachers console him (about 20 minutes); he then attempts the assignments.
>
> **How disruptive or dangerous is the problem behavior(s)?**
> Behavior is not dangerous but is disruptive to class and may have negative social consequences (e.g., other students have already started labeling Randall as a cry baby).

Description of the Antecedents
Identifying Routines: When, where, and with whom are problem behaviors most likely?

Schedule (Times)	Activity	Specific Problem Behavior	Likelihood of Problem Behavior	With Whom Does Problem Occur?
8:30–9:30	Math		Low High ① 2 3 4 5 6	Mrs. Singh
9:30–10:30	Physical Education		① 2 3 4 5 6	Mr. Woods
10:30–11:30	Social Studies	Cries, refuses to do work	1 2 3 4 ⑤ 6	Mrs. Nielsen
11:30–12:00	Lunch		① 2 3 4 5 6	
12:00–12:30	Homeroom		① 2 3 4 5 6	Mr. Sanchez
12:30–1:30	English/Language Arts	Cries, refuses to do work	1 2 3 4 5 ⑥	Mrs. Nielsen
1:30–2:30	Science	Cries, refuses to do work	1 2 ③ 4 5 6	Mrs. Avila
2:30–3:30	Industrial Arts		① 2 3 4 5 6	Mr. Carpenter

(cont.)

FIGURE 8.5. Example of a completed F-BSP teacher interview demonstrating a need for BEP plus modifications for attention-motivated behavior.

Summarize Antecedents (and Setting Events)

> **What situations seem to set off the problem behavior?** (difficult tasks, transitions, structured activities, small-group settings, teacher's request, particular individuals, etc.)
> Classes that require written work. Recent assessments indicate that Randall is capable of completing the work. He is organized, brings materials to class (binder, pencil, paper) and participates in class.
>
> **When is the problem behavior most likely to occur?** (times of day and days of the week)
> During Social Studies, English, and sometimes Science, approximately four to five times per week.
>
> **When is the problem behavior least likely to occur?** (times of day and days of the week)
> During P.E., Industrial Arts, Lunch, Math, and Homeroom.
>
> **Setting Events: Are there specific conditions, events, or activities that make the problem behavior worse?** (missed medication, history of academic failure, conflict at home, missed meals, lack of sleep, history of problems with peers, etc.)
> None identified.

Description of the Consequences

> **What ususally happens after the behavior occurs?** (what is the teacher's reaction, how do other students react, is the student sent to the office, does the student get out of doing work, does the student get in a power struggle, etc.)
> When Randall cries, he is consoled by friends and the teachers, who say "It's all right—you can do it," etc. A couple of times the counselor has come down to try to console Randall. Randall ends up not completing his work.

- - - - - - End of Interview - - - - - -

Step 2: Propose a Testable Explanation

Setting Events	Antecedents	Behaviors	Consequences
	Classes requiring written work (e.g., Social Studies, English)	Randall cries, crosses arms, puts head down, and refuses to do work	Consoling from friends, teachers, and sometimes counselor

Function of the Behavior

For each ABC sequence listed above, why do you think the behavior is occurring? (to get teacher attention, peer attention, desired object/activity, or escape undesirable activity, demand particular people, etc.)

1. <u>When Randall is given a written assignment he cries, crosses his arms, and puts his head down in order</u>
   <u>to gain attention from peers and teachers in the form of consoling (e.g., telling him it will be all right,</u>
   <u>etc.)</u>

How confident are you that your testable explanation is accurate?

Very sure			So-so			Not at all sure
6	⑤		4	3	2	1

FIGURE 8.5. *(cont.)*

poor work completion serves a specific purpose for Randall. It provides a method for obtaining significant attention from both teachers and peers.

In this example, the basic BEP will address some of Randall's attention-motivated behavior. However, the basic BEP may not be sufficient because it does not address Randall's ability to obtain peer attention for inappropriate behavior (other students stop doing their work to look at him, help him, or console him). A modified BEP could include a means for Randall to earn peer attention for appropriate behavior. For example, the classroom could earn an award contingent on Randall's behavior. If Randall completes his assignment and does not cry or become withdrawn, the whole class could earn an extra 5 minutes of recess. In this scenario, students in the classroom would be expected to encourage Randall to meet his goal and to complete his assignment.

Alternatively, Randall may feel too much pressure if the group's reward relies solely on his behavior. The teacher could remove some of this burden with a slight change. The teacher could say that the class will earn an extra recess if everyone in the class finishes their assignment on time. This requirement should have the same impact on Randall's behavior and the behavior of his peers, without putting undue pressure on him alone. Other ways to provide Randall with peer attention may include (1) providing a tangible reinforcer that could be shared with peers (e.g., tokens for the snack bar) upon meeting goals; (2) providing reinforcement to peers for helping Randall to be successful on the BEP; or (3) having him earn an outside-of-classroom activity with peers contingent on successful progress on the BEP.

BEP Plus Modifications for Escape-Motivated Behavior

Finally, Figure 8.6 illustrates how the same behavior, poor work completion, could be an indication of escape-motivated behavior. In this example, according to Mrs. Nielsen, Randall rarely turns in his homework assignments. When Mrs. Nielsen hands out an assignment, Randall will work very slowly, daydream a lot, and not complete his work by the end of the period. Mrs. Nielsen says that the work is not too difficult for Randall. He completes his work perfectly if the task is shortened or if he is told he can read his *Harry Potter* book once his work is completed. At times, when Mrs. Nielsen confronts him about his lack of work completion, he makes rude comments and stomps back to his desk. When Randall is asked to work on a worksheet in class, he announces that he thinks "This class is stupid." The other students rarely attend to Randall's outbursts. If Mrs. Nielsen presses him to complete the assignment in class, he may have a "blowup" in which he throws his books on the floor, rips up the assignment, and yells, "I hate this stupid class." After a blowup, Randall is usually sent to the office, where he is expected to sit calmly for the rest of the class period. A clear outcome of this behavior is that Randall is escaping an aversive situation: doing work in English class. It appears that his behavior is escape-motivated. Randall's math teacher reports similar behavior patterns.

In this case, Randall should benefit from modifications to the BEP that address his escape-motivated behavior. Before a modified BEP can be effective, Randall's teachers and the administrative staff must make a commitment to changing their own reactions to Randall's behavior. His problem behavior can no longer be effective in allowing him to escape an academic task. Randall's teachers must commit to keeping him in class and expecting him to complete his work. If his behavior becomes so disruptive that he *must* be removed from the classroom, then the administrative staff must commit to having him complete his assignments while he is in the office. The inappropriate behavior must first be rendered ineffective. Once Randall no lon-

FUNCTIONAL BEHAVIORAL ASSESSMENT INTERVIEW—TEACHER/STAFF/PARENT

Student name: _Randall_   Age: _13_   Grade: _6_   Date: _12/2/09_

Person(s) interviewed: _Mrs. Nielsen_

Interviewer: _Mr. Jensen_

Student Profile: What is the student good at or what are some strengths that the student brings to school?

Has a good sense of humor, is athletic, and is well liked by other students.

Step 1: Interview Teacher/Staff/Parent
Description of the Behavior

> **What does the problem behavior(s) look like?**
> Randall does not complete class (or homework) but instead sits at his desk, looks out the window, plays with objects. If pressed to do work, will yell, tear up things, and/or throw things.
>
> **How often does the problem behavior(s) occur?**
> Six to seven times a week when homework is due or assignments are given in class that take an extensive amount of time to complete.
>
> **How long does the problem behavior(s) last when it does occur?**
> It can take all period to try to get Randall to do work.
>
> **How disruptive or dangerous is the problem behavior(s)?**
> Behavior is dangerous when he throws objects and is disruptive to the overall flow of classroom activity.

Description of the Antecedents
Identifying Routines: When, where, and with whom are problem behaviors most likely?

Schedule (Times)	Activity	Specific Problem Behavior	Likelihood of Problem Behavior		With Whom Does Problem Occur?
8:30–9:30	Math	Refuses to do work	Low High 1 2 3 4 ⑤ 6		Mrs. Singh
9:30–10:30	Physical Education		① 2 3 4 5 6		Mr. Woods
10:30–11:30	Social Studies	Refuses to do work	1 2 3 4 ⑤ 6		Mrs. Nielsen
11:30–12:00	Lunch		① 2 3 4 5 6		
12:00–12:30	Homeroom		① 2 3 4 5 6		Mr. Sanchez
12:30–1:30	English/Language Arts	Refuses to do work	1 2 3 4 5 ⑥		Mrs. Nielsen
1:30–2:30	Science	Refuses to do work	1 2 ③ 4 5 6		Mrs. Avila
2:30–3:30	Industrial Arts		① 2 3 4 5 6		Mr. Carpenter

(cont.)

FIGURE 8.6. Example of a completed F-BSP teacher interview demonstrating a need for BEP plus modifications for escape-motivated behavior.

Summarize Antecedents (and Setting Events)

> **What situations seem to set off the problem behavior?** (difficult tasks, transitions, structured activities, small-group settings, teacher's request, particular individuals, etc.)
> When asked to do work or turn in homework, particularly lengthy assignments
>
> **When is the problem behavior most likely to occur?** (times of day and days of the week)
> During Social Studies, Math, English, and sometimes Science
>
> **When is the problem behavior least likely to occur?** (times of day and days of the week)
> During P.E., Industrial Arts, Lunch, and Homeroom.
>
> **Setting Events: Are there specific conditions, events, or activities that make the problem behavior worse?** (missed medication, history of academic failure, conflict at home, missed meals, lack of sleep, history of problems with peers, etc.)
> None identified.

Description of the Consequences

> **What ususally happens after the behavior occurs?** (what is the teacher's reaction, how do other students react, is the student sent to the office, does the student get out of doing work, does the student get in a power struggle, etc.)
> When Randall refuses to do work, he will sit, look out the window, etc., and when pressed to do work he will yell ("This is stupid!") and at times throw books and tear up assignments. Sometimes he is sent to the office. He is able to get out of doing work when he engages in these behaviors.

- - - - - - End of Interview - - - - - -

Step 2: Propose a Testable Explanation

Setting Events	Antecedents	Behaviors	Consequences
	Instructed to do work	Refuses to do work and yells/throws objects if pressed to do work	Does not complete work Ultimately sent to office

Function of the Behavior

For each ABC sequence listed above, why do you think the behavior is occurring? (to get teacher attention, peer attention, desired object/activity, or escape undesirable activity, demand particular people, etc.)

1. When Randall is given an assignment, he looks out the window, plays with objects, and ultimately ends up escaping the work that was required for the class.

How confident are you that your testable explanation is accurate?

Very sure			So-so			Not at all sure
6	⑤		4	3	2	1

FIGURE 8.6. *(cont.)*

ger receives a reward (escape from work) for inappropriate behavior, a modified BEP can be introduced that allows him to earn personally meaningful rewards for meeting his BEP goals. Rewards should be determined through a discussion with Randall. Example rewards might include (1) leaving social studies class 15 minutes early, once a week; (2) working as a library helper once a week during math class; or (3) being excused from one English assignment per week. Each of these strategies allows Randall to escape some work in math, social studies, and English, in exchange for demonstrating appropriate, not inappropriate, behavior.

Figures 8.7–8.9 illustrate the same interview information in a different format. This structured interview is called the Functional Assessment Checklist for Teachers and Staff (FACTS). The FACTS is quite similar to the F-BSP Protocol interviews. The two instruments differ somewhat in format, but both are used to gather similar information. Either instrument is a time-efficient method to determine simple strategies to use to modify a student's BEP.

The BEP Support Plan illustrated in Figure 8.10 demonstrates how the information gathered in the simple FBA interview can be converted into specific strategies for the modified BEP.

Blank copies of the BEP Support Plan, F-BSP Protocol Teacher/Staff/Parent Interview, and the FACTS, along with instructions for completing the interviews, are included in Appendices G.2, G.3, and G.4, respectively.

BEP STUDENTS WITH AN INDIVIDUALIZED EDUCATION PLAN

As students are identified for the BEP, the behavior support team may find that a large proportion of these students are receiving special education services. This is quite common for students with behavioral challenges warranting BEP intervention. Each student receiving special education services will have an individualized education plan (IEP). The behavior support and IEP teams should consider the linkage between these two programs to ensure that the best interests of each student are served. The two teams should consider the following issues:

1. The BEP should not contradict the student's IEP.
2. The BEP should support the IEP.
3. If a student has an IEP goal for behavioral issues, the BEP alone will not be adequate to address that IEP goal.

The BEP is a Tier II intervention implemented at the group level. Students who are on a basic BEP go through the same program and have the same goals. In contrast, an IEP is individualized to the needs of each individual student. The IEP is typically more comprehensive than a BEP. An IEP for a student with behavioral goals could, as an example, list the following types of services and strategies: (1) half-hour of anger management class per week with the school counselor; (2) desk placed in front of the classroom, nearest the teacher; (3) early dismissal between class periods; and (4) BEP intervention. In other words, the basic BEP is only one component of the IEP. It should not be used as the sole strategy for addressing the behavioral problems of a student with an IEP for behavioral issues.

(text continues on page 123)

FACTS—Part A

Step 1

Student/Grade: <u>Randall—6th</u>   Date: <u>12/6/09</u>

Interviewer: <u>Mr. Jensen</u>   Respondent(s): <u>Mrs. Nielsen</u>

Step 2 **Student Profile: Please identify at least three strengths or contributions the student brings to school.**

<u>Athletic, liked by peers, and good sense of humor</u>

Step 3 **Problem Behavior(s): Identify problem behaviors**

___ Tardy	___ Inappropriate language	___ Disruptive	___ Theft
___ Unresponsive	___ Fight/physical aggression	___ Insubordination	___ Vandalism
___ Withdrawn	___ Verbal harassment	_X_ Work not done	___ Other _____

Describe problem behavior: <u>Randall forgets to bring his materials (e.g., binder, pencil, paper) to class</u>
<u>and often forgets his homework.</u>

Step 4 **Identifying Routines: Where, when, and with whom are problem behaviors are most likely?**

Schedule (Times)	Activity	With Whom Does Problem Occur?	Likelihood of Problem Behavior	Specific Problem Behavior
8:30–9:30	Math	Mr. Singh	Low High 1 2 3 4 ⑤ 6	Unorganized/ forgets homework
9:30–10:30	Physical Education	Mr. Woods	① 2 3 4 5 6	
10:30–11:30	Social Studies	Mrs. Nielsen	1 2 3 4 5 ⑥	Unorganized/ forgets homework
11:30–12:00	Lunch		① 2 3 4 5 6	
12:00–12:30	Homeroom	Mr. Sanchez	① 2 3 4 5 6	
12:30–1:30	English/Language Arts	Mrs. Nielsen	1 2 3 4 5 ⑥	Unorganized/ forgets homework
1:30–2:30	Science	Mrs. Avila	1 2 3 ④ 5 6	
2:30–3:30	Industrial Arts	Mr. Carpenter	1 ② 3 4 5 6	

Step 5 Select one to three routines for further assessment. Select routines based on (1) similarity of activities (conditions) with ratings of 4, 5, or 6 and (2) similarity of problem behavior(s). Complete the FACTS—Part B for each routine identified.

(cont.)

FIGURE 8.7. Example of a completed FACTS teacher interview demonstrating a need for BEP plus academic supports.

FACTS—Part B

Step 1 Student/Grade: _Randall—6th_   Date: _12/6/09_

Interviewer: _Mr. Jensen_   Respondent(s): _Mrs. Nielsen_

<u>Step 2</u> **Routine/Activities/Context: Which routine (only one) from the FACTS—Part A is assessed?**

Routine/Activities/Context	Problem Behavior
Classes that require homework and organization with materials.	Does not complete work

Step 3 **Provide more detail about the problem behavior(s):**

What does the problem behavior(s) look like? Incomplete and missing assignments; Randall forgets to bring his materials (e.g., binder, pencil, paper) to class and often forgets his homework.

How often does the problem behavior(s) occur? Assignments are missing on a weekly basis in Math, Social Stuidies, and English.

How long does the problem behavior(s) last when it does occur? If Randall forgets his materials and homework it can disrupt the whole period because he is not ready to go over the homework and is unprepared for the new lesson.

What is the intensity/level of danger of the problem behavior(s)? Behavior is not dangerous but is disruptive to his academic performance. At risk for being retained.

Step 4 **What are the events that predict when the problem behavior(s) will occur?**

Related Issues (Setting Events)		Environmental Features	
___illness	Other:_____	___reprimand/correction	_X_ structured activity
___drug use	_____	___physical demands	___unstructured time
___negative social	_____	___socially isolated	___tasks too boring
___conflict at home	_____	___with peers	___activity too long
___academic failure	_____	___other	___tasks too difficult

Step 5 **What consequences are most likely to maintain the problem behavior(s)?**

Things That Are Obtained		Things Avoided or Escaped From	
___adult attention	Other:_Homework incomplete_	___hard tasks	Other:_____
___peer attention	_and poor grades_	___reprimands	_____
___preferred activity	_____	___peer negatives	_____
___money/things	_____	___physical effort	_____

Step 6 **What current efforts have been used to control the problem behavior?**

Strategies for Preventing Problem Behavior		Consequences for Problem Behavior	
___schedule change	Other:_____	_X_ reprimand	Other:_____
_X_ seating change	_____	___office referral	_____
___curriculum change	_____	___detention	_____

SUMMARY OF BEHAVIOR

Step 7 **Identify the summary that will be used to build a plan of behavior support.**

Setting Events and Predictors	Problem Behavior(s)	Maintaining Consequence(s)
Classes requiring organization/ Homework (e.g., Math, Social Studies)	1. Lack of homework 2. Lack of materials	Poor grades

How confident are you that the Summary of Behavior is accurate?

Not very confident					Very confident
1	2	3	4	⑤	6

FIGURE 8.7. *(cont.)*

FACTS—Part A

Step 1

Student/Grade: Randall—6th   Date: 12/6/09

Interviewer: Mr. Jensen   Respondent(s): Mrs. Nielsen

Step 2 **Student Profile: Please identify at least three strengths or contributions the student brings to school.**

Athletic, liked by peers, and good sense of humor

Step 3 **Problem Behavior(s): Identify problem behaviors**

___ Tardy	___ Inappropriate language	___ Disruptive	___ Theft
___ Unresponsive	___ Fight/physical aggression	___ Insubordination	___ Vandalism
X Withdrawn	___ Verbal harassment	X Work not done	___ Other _____

Describe problem behavior: Randall becomes teary-eyed and refuses to do work (sits with arms crossed, head down) when given a written assignment.

Step 4 **Identifying Routines: Where, when, and with whom are problem behaviors are most likely?**

Schedule (Times)	Activity	With Whom Does Problem Occur?	Likelihood of Problem Behavior	Specific Problem Behavior
8:30–9:30	Math	Mr. Singh	Low High ① 2 3 4 5 6	Cries, refuses to do work
9:30–10:30	Physical Education	Mr. Woods	① 2 3 4 5 6	
10:30–11:30	Social Studies	Mrs. Nielsen	1 2 3 4 ⑤ 6	Cries, refuses to do work
11:30–12:00	Lunch		① 2 3 4 5 6	
12:00–12:30	Homeroom	Mr. Sanchez	① 2 3 4 5 6	
12:30–1:30	English/Language Arts	Mrs. Nielsen	1 2 3 4 5 ⑥	Cries, refuses to do work
1:30–2:30	Science	Mrs. Avila	1 ② 3 4 5 6	Cries, refuses to do work
2:30–3:30	Industrial Arts	Mr. Carpenter	① 2 3 4 5 6	

Step 5 Select one to three routines for further assessment. Select routines based on (1) similarity of activities (conditions) with ratings of 4, 5, or 6 and (2) similarity of problem behavior(s). Complete the FACTS—Part B for each routine identified.

(cont.)

FIGURE 8.8. Example of a completed FACTS teacher interview demonstrating a need for BEP plus modifications for attention-motivated behavior.

FACTS—Part B

Step 1 Student/Grade: Randall—6th   Date: 12/6/09

Interviewer: Mr. Jensen   Respondent(s): Mrs. Nielsen

Step 2 **Routine/Activities/Context: Which routine (only one) from the FACTS—Part A is assessed?**

Routine/Activities/Context	Problem Behavior
Classes that require written work	Does not complete work and cries

Step 3 **Provide more detail about the problem behavior(s):**

What does the problem behavior(s) look like? Classes that require written work. Recent assessments indicate that Randall is capable of completing the work. He is organized, brings materials to class (binder, pencil, paper) and participates in class.

How often does the problem behavior(s) occur? During Social Studies, English, and sometimes Science, approximately four to five times per week.

How long does the problem behavior(s) last when it does occur? Randall cries and refuses to do work until friends and teachers console him (about 20 minutes), he then attempts the assignments.

What is the intensity/level of danger of the problem behavior(s)? Behavior is not dangerous but is disruptive to class and may have negative social consequences (e.g., other students have already started labeling Randall as a cry baby).

Step 4 **What are the events that predict when the problem behavior(s) will occur?**

Related Issues (Setting Events)		Environmental Features	
___ illness	Other:_____	___ reprimand/correction	X structured activity
___ drug use	_____	___ physical demands	___ unstructured time
___ negative social	_____	___ socially isolated	___ tasks too boring
___ conflict at home	_____	X with peers	___ activity too long
___ academic failure	_____	X other writing activity	___ tasks too difficult

Step 5 **What consequences are most likely to maintain the problem behavior(s)?**

Things That Are Obtained		Things Avoided or Escaped From	
X adult attention	Other:_____	___ hard tasks	Other:_____
X peer attention	_____	___ reprimands	_____
___ preferred activity	_____	___ peer negatives	_____
___ money/things	_____	___ physical effort	_____

Step 6 **What current efforts have been used to control the problem behavior?**

Strategies for Preventing Problem Behavior		Consequences for Problem Behavior	
___ schedule change	Other:_____	X reprimand	Other:_____
___ seating change	_____	___ office referral	_____
X curriculum change	_____	___ detention	_____

SUMMARY OF BEHAVIOR

Step 7 **Identify the summary that will be used to build a plan of behavior support.**

Setting Events and Predictors	Problem Behavior(s)	Maintaining Consequence(s)
Classes requiring written work (e.g., Social Studies, English)	Randall cries, crosses arms, puts head down, and refuses to do work	Consoling from friends, teachers, and sometimes counselor

How confident are you that the Summary of Behavior is accurate?

Not very confident					Very confident
1	2	3	4	⑤	6

FIGURE 8.8. *(cont.)*

FACTS—Part A

Step 1

Student/Grade: Randall—6th   Date: 12/6/09

Interviewer: Mr. Jensen   Respondent(s): Mrs. Nielsen

Step 2 **Student Profile: Please identify at least three strengths or contributions the student brings to school.**

Athletic, liked by peers, and good sense of humor

Step 3 **Problem Behavior(s): Identify problem behaviors**

___ Tardy	___ Inappropriate language	X Disruptive	___ Theft
___ Unresponsive	___ Fight/physical aggression	___ Insubordination	___ Vandalism
___ Withdrawn	X Verbal harassment	X Work not done	___ Other _____
	X Verbally inappropriate	___ Self-injury	

Describe problem behavior: _Randall does not complete class (or homework) but instead sits at his desk, looks out the window and plays with objects. If pressed to do work, will yell, tear up things, and/or throw things._

Step 4 **Identifying Routines: Where, when, and with whom are problem behaviors are most likely?**

Schedule (Times)	Activity	With Whom Does Problem Occur?	Likelihood of Problem Behavior	Specific Problem Behavior
8:30–9:30	Math	Mr. Singh	Low High 1 2 3 4 ⑤ 6	Refuses to do work
9:30–10:30	Physical Education	Mr. Woods	① 2 3 4 5 6	
10:30–11:30	Social Studies	Mrs. Nielsen	1 2 3 4 ⑤ 6	Refuses to do work
11:30–12:00	Lunch		① 2 3 4 5 6	
12:00–12:30	Homeroom	Mr. Sanchez	① 2 3 4 5 6	
12:30–1:30	English/Language Arts	Mrs. Nielsen	1 2 3 4 5 ⑥	Refuses to do work
1:30–2:30	Science	Mrs. Avila	1 2 ③ 4 5 6	Refuses to do work
2:30–3:30	Industrial Arts	Mr. Carpenter	① 2 3 4 5 6	

Step 5 Select one to three routines for further assessment. Select routines based on (1) similarity of activities (conditions) with ratings of 4, 5, or 6 and (2) similarity of problem behavior(s). Complete the FACTS—Part B for each routine identified.

(cont.)

FIGURE 8.9. Example of a completed FACTS teacher interview demonstrating a need for BEP plus modifications for escape-motivated behavior.

FACTS—Part B

Step 1 Student/Grade: _Randall—6th_   Date: _12/6/09_

Interviewer: _Mr. Jensen_   Respondent(s): _Mrs. Nielsen_

Step 2 **Routine/Activities/Context: Which routine (only one) from the FACTS—Part A is assessed?**

Routine/Activities/Context	Problem Behavior
Classes that require homework and/or lengthy class assignments	Does not complete work, inappropriate language, throwing objects

Step 3 **Provide more detail about the problem behavior(s):**

What does the problem behavior(s) look like? Randall does not complete class (or homework) but instead sits at his desk, looks out the window and plays with objects. If pressed to do work, he will yell, tear up things, and/or throw things.

How often does the problem behavior(s) occur? Six or seven times a week when homework is due or assignments are given in class that take an extensive amount of time to complete.

How long does the problem behavior(s) last when it does occur? It can take all period to try to get Randall to do work.

What is the intensity/level of danger of the problem behavior(s)? Behavior is dangerous when he throws objects and is disruptive to the overall flow of classroom activity.

Step 4 **What are the events that predict when the problem behavior(s) will occur?**

Related Issues (Setting Events)		Environmental Features	
___ illness	Other:_____	___ reprimand/correction	X structured activity
___ drug use	_____	___ physical demands	___ unstructured time
___ negative social	_____	___ socially isolated	___ tasks too boring
___ conflict at home	_____	X with peers	X activity too long
___ academic failure	_____	X Other: Asked to hand in homework	___ tasks too difficult

Step 5 **What consequences are most likely to maintain the problem behavior(s)?**

Things That Are Obtained		Things Avoided or Escaped From	
___ adult attention	Other:_____	___ hard tasks	Other: _structured and/or_
___ peer attention	_____	___ reprimands	_lengthy tasks_
___ preferred activity	_____	___ peer negatives	_____
___ money/things	_____	___ physical effort	_____

Step 6 **What current efforts have been used to control the problem behavior?**

Strategies for Preventing Problem Behavior		Consequences for Problem Behavior	
X schedule change	Other:_____	X reprimand	Other:_____
___ seating change	_____	___ office referral	_____
X curriculum change	_____	___ detention	_____

SUMMARY OF BEHAVIOR

Step 7 **Identify the summary that will be used to build a plan of behavior support.**

Setting Events and Predictors	Problem Behavior(s)	Maintaining Consequence(s)
Instructed to do work	Refuses to do work and yells/throws objects if pressed to do work	Does not complete work Ultimately sent to office

How confident are you that the Summary of Behavior is accurate?

Not very confident					Very confident
1	2	3	4	⑤	6

FIGURE 8.9. *(cont.)*

BEP Support Plan

Name: _Randall Prima_   Date of support request: _1/6/10_   Grade: _6th_

Parent's name: _Alice Prima_   Parent's phone no: _504.876.5432_

Requested by: _Mrs. Nielsen (Social Studies teacher)_

Reason for request: _Behavior has not improved though he's been on BEP for 1 month already._

Functional Behavioral Assessment Activites

Step 1: Gather Information (Give dates of completion)

Parent Contact _1/8/10_   Staffing _1/13/10_   Observation (optional) _____

FBA Interview _1/10/10_   Student Interview (optional) _1/10/10_

IEP: ___ Yes _X_ No   No. of office referrals: _13_   No. of absences: _6_

Step 2: Propose a Summary Statement of the Problem

What sets off the problem?	What are the problems?	Why are they happening?
Instructed to do assignment (especially written work)	Refuses to do work and yells/throws objects if pressed to do work.	Does not complete work. Ultimately sent to office and thereby gets out of class and the assignment.

Step 3: Propose Appropriate BEP Options

☐ Basic BEP   ☒ Modified BEP   ☐ Individualized Support   ☐ Other

(cont.)

FIGURE 8.10. Example of a completed BEP Support Plan.

Design Support Plan

Step 4: Conduct BEP Team Meetings to Determine Student Goal and Design Plan

Student Goal: Randall will complete assignments in class without disruption to himself, the teacher, or his peers.

Additional Supports	When	Where	Who Responsible
BEP will be monitored by his football coach	Twice daily	Gym office	Mr. Reynolds
Randall will have opportunity to earn personally meaningful rewards on daily and weekly basis after meeting BEP goals	Daily or weekly, dependent on goal / reinforcer set by Mr. Reynolds	Varies	Mr. Reynolds

Step 5: Conduct Review Meetings and Use Student Monitoring Form to Monitor Progress

BEP Student Monitoring Form

Student Name: Randall   Facilitator Name: Mr. Reynolds

Student Goal: Randall will complete assignments in class without disruption to himself, the teacher, or his peers

Date	Additional Supports Completed	To do next • Continue • Modify • Monitor	Student's Progress
1/20/10	Mr. Reynolds has become Randall's BEP facilitator	Continue	It seems to have improved his consistency in turning in DPRs.
1/27/10	Randall has earned several personally meaningful reinforcers (e.g., time to be office aide, 10 minutes free time in gym) as a result of meeting daily goal	Modify—increase goal to 80% of points. Gradually fade from daily reward to weekly reward.	Randall has been meeting daily goal (75% of points). Behavior is improved. Increase in assignment completion.

FIGURE 8.10. *(cont.)*

Is a modified BEP with individualized goals sufficient to address an IEP behavioral goal? This question can be answered only on a case-by-case basis. The adequacy of the IEP is dependent on the needs of the child. If the behavioral needs of a child with an IEP behavioral goal are adequately addressed and reduced by a modified BEP, then it is reasonable to assume that the BEP is adequate and sufficient. This is, however, unlikely. A student who receives special education services for behavioral issues typically has complex needs that require more than a simple, Tier II intervention. When a BEP is included in a student's IEP, we recommend that it be used as one part of a comprehensive plan and not as the only strategy for addressing the student's behavioral needs.

Communication between the BEP and IEP Teams

It is essential that all of the individuals or teams who work to resolve the behavioral issues of a student work in concert, not in conflict. At the very least, the behavior support team should have access to a list of students who have an IEP for behavioral goals. Any time a student on an IEP is considered for placement on the BEP, an IEP team member for that student should be invited to the behavior support team meeting. The IEP team member can communicate the behavior support team's suggestions to the rest of the IEP team.

If the IEP team chooses to incorporate the BEP into the student's IEP, they must hold an IEP meeting and make the appropriate modifications. However, placement on the BEP does not always necessitate a change in the student's IEP. A student may be placed on the BEP without any changes to the IEP. In such a case, the BEP is a service that the student receives through the school, but it is not a required part of the student's IEP contract. Placement on the BEP necessitates a change in the IEP only if (1) participation in the BEP precludes participation in some other aspect of the student's current IEP; (2) participation in the BEP creates a change in the student's IEP behavioral goals; or (3) the IEP team chooses to list the BEP as one strategy for addressing the student's IEP goal.

To enhance communication between the behavior support team and the special education team, we strongly suggest that the behavior support team include at least one special education teacher. This teacher will attend behavior support team meetings as well as special education team meetings. When a student comes up for discussion with either group, the special education teacher can act as representative, communicating information between both teams.

Communication between the behavior support team and special education team can be further enhanced by using the following strategies:

1. Keep a copy of the student's IEP face page in his or her BEP file. Thus, if a student comes up for "priority" discussion, the BEP team will have easy access to relevant IEP information.
2. If a student is slated for "priority" discussion at the behavior support team meeting, invite the student's special education case manager to the meeting.
3. If a BEP student has an upcoming IEP meeting, invite a behavior support team member to attend the meeting to share information on the student's BEP goals and progress. If the person is unable to attend, ensure open lines of communication so that the IEP team can have easy access to the student's IEP data.

CHAPTER 9

High School Implementation of the BEP

Jessica Swain-Bradway and Robert H. Horner

The BEP can be implemented with precision and success in high school. The basic functions of the BEP are to (1) establish a predictable daily structure; (2) increase the frequency and contingency of adult feedback; and (3) improve the consistency of home–school communication to have relevance for students in high school. High school implementation of the BEP is more complex than middle school or elementary school implementation, because (1) students function at a developmental level where peer attention is relatively more reinforcing than adult attention; (2) students are expected to self-manage both their social and academic behaviors; (3) the greater physical size of high schools makes coordination among adults more complex; and (4) many adults in high schools do not view the development or management of students' social behaviors as a responsibility or priority (Bohanon-Edmonson, Flannery, Eber, & Sugai, 2005).

The combined effect of these variables necessitates modifications to the BEP to fit the high school culture. First, the social supports within the high school BEP need to be modified to emphasize self-management and link students with those specific adults they identify as being "cool," or reinforcing. Second, due to the central role of academics in high schools, social supports must be complemented with academic support that is sufficient to maintain academic engagement. The academic supports needed to accomplish this goal include development of a small number of core academic skills (e.g., use of academic planner, notebook organization and maintenance, test taking, and study skills) and ongoing assistance with daily academic demands (Lenz & Deshler, 1998; Flannery, McGrath Kato, Fenning, & Bohanon, in press; Swanson & Deshler, 2003).

In this chapter, we outline an approach for applying basic BEP practices with the enhanced social and academic elements that make the BEP functional at the high school level. First, the conceptual and organizational similarities between the elementary and middle school BEP and

Jessica Swain-Bradway, PhD, is a Research Associate, University of Oregon, Special Education, Eugene, Oregon.

the high school BEP model are presented. Next, the logic for adapting the BEP to meet the needs of high school students is presented. Following the overview of the adaptations, specific steps to achieve these adaptations are outlined. Finally, current efforts to use this adapted BEP approach in high schools in the Pacific Northwest are described and preliminary results are summarized.

RELEVANCE OF BEP PRINCIPLES FOR HIGH SCHOOL STUDENTS

The core behavioral principles of the BEP extend logically to the high school setting. Systematic adult interaction and well-defined behavioral goals provide increased structure to a student's day as he or she moves from classroom to classroom. The BEP prompts an increase in positive, contingent feedback from multiple adults, thereby (1) supporting students' ability to navigate different classroom expectations and (2) increasing students' connection to school (Crone et al., 2004). The home–school connection is strengthened through increased daily communication. For high school students, these components are as pertinent as they are for elementary or middle school students.

In addition, many of the administrative features of the BEP at the elementary and middle school level are appropriate for implementation of the BEP in high school. Establishing screening procedures and fading protocols, utilizing data for decision making, and close monitoring of student progress are elements that serve to establish the systemwide capacity of the BEP (Hawken & Horner, 2003). The weekly and quarterly BEP administrative processes are necessary for implementation of an efficient BEP at any level: (1) summarizing data for each BEP student; (2) prioritizing students for behavior team meetings; (3) using data to determine if a student's BEP should be continued, modified, or ended; (4) awarding reinforcers to students who attain specific goals; (5) discussing potential new BEP candidates; and (6) assigning organizational tasks to relevant staff members (Bohanon-Edmonson et al., 2005). Updating staff members on student progress is another important component of the BEP for elementary and middle schools that extends to the high school setting. Teachers and staff need to know how many students are participating in the BEP, as well as how those students are progressing.

Other BEP features may have more developmental relevance for high school students. Features such as the establishment of self-management and self-regulation skills and the expansion of positive relationships with adults are components that mimic workplace demands once students graduate from high school. Establishing positive relationships with adults is notably important to high school students who are at risk for dropping out of school. *High schools that report a high proportion of supportive teachers cut the probability of dropping out in half for their students* (Croninger & Lee, 2001).

The conceptual logic underlying the BEP has applicability for supporting the needs of high school students. However, important developmental and contextual differences should be considered in the implementation of the BEP in high school. The following sections outline the basic adaptations recommended for the high school BEP model:

1. The combination of academic and social supports.
2. The participation of students in data review, action planning, and adaptations.
3. Target population for the BEP.

BEP PLUS ACADEMIC SUPPORTS: COHESIVE SUPPORT FOR HIGH SCHOOL STUDENTS

The defining difference of the BEP in high school settings addresses the connection between academic performance and problem behavior (Morrison, Anthony, Storino, & Dillon, 2001; Roeser & Eccles, 2000). The high school BEP combines social and academic supports for students demonstrating Tier II behavioral needs. Figure 9.1 provides a summary linking the core elements associated with effective implementation of the BEP within a high school. We review each of these elements briefly and later describe, in more detail, how core adaptations may be accomplished.

Schoolwide Supports, Referral for BEP

High school implementation of the BEP begins, as in elementary and middle school, with the adoption of schoolwide behavior and academic supports (Crone et al., 2004). Within the framework of schoolwide behavior and academic supports, the broad social culture of the school is expected to be predictable, consistent, positive, and safe. The academic culture of the school is expected to rely on evidence-based curricula, well-planned instruction at appropriate intensity, and sufficient progress monitoring to ensure early identification of students at risk (Horner, Sugai, Todd, & Lewis-Palmer, 2005). When a student experiences either social or academic risk he or she is identified early and referred for assistance. The referral process is efficient, resulting in rapid access to academic support, behavior support, or both.

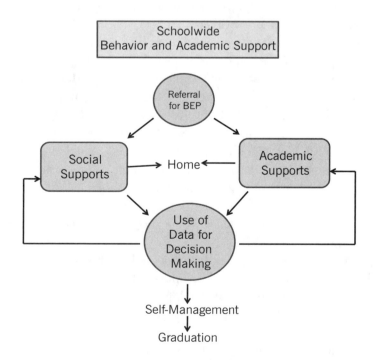

FIGURE 9.1. The high school BEP cycle.

Social Supports

Many of the features of the high school BEP social support are similar to characteristics of social support for elementary and middle school students: (1) a morning check-in with an adult, (2) ongoing performance feedback from adults at predictable times throughout the day, (3) an afternoon check-out with an adult, (4) a formal process for linking home–school feedback to the student, and (5) the critical features of the DPR. The high school BEP uses data on student performance to assess impact of supports and guide adaptation, as is done in elementary and middle school versions of the BEP.

The difference in the social supports of the high school BEP lies in the extent to which the student him- or herself participates in data review, action planning, and the design of adaptations. Students should be actively involved in weekly or twice-monthly reviews of their progress on the BEP, assignment completion, grades, and attendance. The BEP coordinator schedules and facilitates the initial progress reviews. As students become fluent in identifying patterns of personal progress at or above goal (80%), the BEP coordinator supportively scaffolds a shift, through modeling and practice, to a self-managed program in which the student is continuously reviewing his or her own behavior and creating specific goals to increase his or her academic and social successes.

As the formal feedback process of the high school BEP is faded out, an informal, more efficient, and increasingly positive process takes its place. Just as with the elementary version of the BEP, teacher feedback can be gradually faded so the student is self-scoring and then checking his or her self-score with the teacher. It may also be appropriate during the fading process to provide only a morning check-in for the student to provide a reminder of the school expectations as they apply to social and academic behaviors. The student becomes fluent in self-management activities and is able to recruit feedback from adults within the "natural" contexts of the school setting.

Due to the aforementioned contextual complexities of the high school environment, this focus on self-management extends beyond the capacity of the brief, daily social support cycle of the BEP. While schoolwide expectations can be extended to specific academic behaviors if students do not possess the skills necessary to engage in positive academic behaviors, the reminders are not functional. For example, "Be responsible" is exemplified not only through social behaviors, such as "Keep your work area clean," but also through specific academic behaviors, such as "Turn in homework on time." In order to turn in homework on time, a student must know (1) assignment details (page number, number of problems, etc.), (2) when the homework is due, and (3) the protocol for handing in homework within the specific classroom. Explicitly providing academic supports, by teaching and practicing organizational skills, creates a cohesive program of support necessary for high school students who are at risk of school failure.

Academic Supports

A defining component of high school BEP implementation is the combination of academic and social supports. While combining academic and social supports may be useful at any grade level, the importance of linking academic supports to the social feedback provided by the BEP is especially important in high school. *Our preliminary findings with the high school BEP suggest that few students (e.g., less than 10%) should participate in the social support component of high school BEP without also receiving the academic support component.* For high school students to remain engaged in academic efforts, they need to avoid frequent punishers (e.g., reprimands, failure, public display of incompetence). Academic supports need not only to address instructional goals, but also to provide the assistance that allows students to engage in academic efforts without frequent punishment. This is no simple goal, given that success in high school is contingent upon students having the skills to master increasingly intense academic demands, such as multichapter midterms, multicomponent class projects, summarizing and synthesizing entire novels, and so on. Academic support in high school should focus specifically on assisting students to be sufficiently successful so that they remain engaged in academic activities. Academic supports that help achieve this goal include (1) basic study skills to remain organized, planful, and efficient; and (2) the daily supports required to meet immediate academic demands, such as homework.

Explicitly teaching academic skills that focus on organizing academic demands can have a dramatic impact on student success. In a 2003 meta-analysis by Swanson and Deshler, teaching organization skills alone was found to contribute to a large percentage (16%) of the increase in positive general education outcomes for students with learning disabilities. Adding a homework assistance component to a BEP intervention can moderate the difficulty of academic tasks through subject matter support. For example, if students on the BEP have time dedicated each day, or a few times each week, to the completion of homework with the assistance of an adult, they are more likely to hand in accurate homework in a timely manner.

Home Component

As with the elementary and middle school BEP, the home component of the DPR is intended to encourage consistent home–school collaboration (Crone et al., 2004). The home–school component is more flexible with the high school BEP. Students who are unable to secure a home signature, for a variety of reasons (personal safety, estrangement, etc.) identify an adult with whom they have a supportive connection in the school. This adult "stands in" for the family contact and provides the home signature for the student. The home component flexibility extends the network of supportive adults within the school environment for the student.

STUDENT PARTICIPATION IN THE HIGH SCHOOL BEP

A high school BEP needs to effectively combine social and academic supports in a way that (1) systematically encourages self-management and self-regulation, and (2) reflects the interests and needs of the participating students. *The systematic encouragement of self-management and self-regulation should be reflected in every aspect of the high school BEP.* Active student participation in designing, implementing, and evaluating a BEP intervention requires the consideration of (1) the developmental needs of teenaged students and (2) the reinforcing quality of providing students with choices. Systematically incorporating opportunities for students to participate in the management of their high school BEP functions to increase their opportunities to practice self-regulation skills and to increase school engagement. High school students must be actively engaged in deciding to participate in the BEP, identifying problem behaviors, creating academic and social goals and action plans, monitoring progress, and making adaptation decisions. Increasing school engagement is especially important for students who have been marginalized by academic failure or problem behaviors (Sinclair et al., 1998).

The ability of a teacher to meaningfully engage students in academic activities is intimately related to his or her knowledge of the students and their families (Kea & Utley, 1998; Klump & McNeir, 2005). The teacher providing instruction for the academic component of high school BEP must know the students well enough to incorporate their interests and strengths into the learning activities. Connecting students' outside interests to school activities further increases school engagement.

TARGET POPULATION FOR THE HIGH SCHOOL BEP

The BEP plus academic supports (high school BEP) can effectively address the needs of students in all high school grades, but may be particularly important for freshman and sophomore students. There are two reasons for targeting students in the first 2 years of high school. First, a majority of high school students decide whether to stay in school or drop out soon after entering high school (Hertzog & Morgan, 1999; Mizelle & Irvin, 2000). Second, the transition from middle to high school can pose considerable difficulties for students who struggled with academic and social success in middle school (Chinien & Boutin, 2001; Forgan & Vaughn, 2000; McIntosh, Flannery, Sugai, Braun, & Cochrane, 2008; Newman, Lohman, Newman, Myers, & Smith, 2000). Students transitioning to high school need to effectively navigate numerous contingencies, including graduation requirements, multiple chapter exams, long-term projects, teacher and content-related expectations that vary by class period, and the relatively greater size of a high school campus (McIntosh et al., 2008). Choosing freshman for the high school BEP reduces some of the difficulties associated with transitioning, while at the same time it increases the probability that students will be equipped to meet the academic and social challenges early in their high school career.

In summary, the BEP for high school students:

1. Effectively combines academic and social supports.
2. Incorporates the interests and developmental needs of high school-age students into learning activities for core academic skills.
3. Targets freshman and sophomore students to minimize the length of time that a student struggles with academic and or social difficulties.

THE HIGH SCHOOL BEP MODEL

The following sections describe, in more detail, how the core adaptations of the high school BEP may be put into practice. Social support and academic support cycles are explained. Evaluation data for a high school located in the Pacific Northwestern United States are then presented. Finally, future considerations for practice are provided.

Referral and Placement

Establishing communication between middle schools and a high school is central to providing continuous support for students transitioning into the high school setting. Students identified for extended school year or summer school between their eighth- and ninth-grade years are excellent candidates for inclusion in the high school BEP. If this information is not available, a clearly defined referral protocol for Tier II supports is necessary to ensure (1) a match between the function of problem behavior and the intervention; (2) prompt implementation of services to decrease the probability of future failures; and (3) written documentation of student supports for accountability purposes. Freshman and sophomore students demonstrating the following Tier II problem behaviors should be considered for inclusion in the high school BEP:

- A grade of D or F, in two to four classes, due to missing assignments or low test scores.
- Minor-to-moderate disruptive behaviors: (1) talk-outs; (2) off-task behavior during academics by drawing, text messaging, or not attending to the teacher.
- Attendance issues such as frequently skipping classes or absences from school, both excused and unexcused.
- Office discipline referrals at a rate of two to three referrals within the first 3 months of school.

The nomination documentation should include the following information:

- Student demographics, including strengths.
- Special education status.
- Number of suspensions received during the current school year.
- An estimate of the student's percentage of homework and class work, as well as grades on tests within the referring teacher's classroom.
- Top three problem behaviors.
- Previous classroom interventions implemented to support positive behaviors.
- The effectiveness of those interventions.
- The teacher's best guess as to why the student continues to engage in problem behavior (i.e., function of behavior).

The high school BEP alone will not provide sufficient support for students displaying Tier III level, or crisis, problem behaviors. The nomination process must include options for immediate support for students who are identified as being in crisis or who are engaging in severe problem behavior such as extreme aggression, violence toward others, or substance abuse.

Once a student has been referred by school personnel for Tier II supports, a behavior support team within the high school must:

1. Review the referral.
2. Determine if more information is needed, such as additional grades, test scores, and ODR records.
3. Determine if the high school BEP is appropriate in meeting student needs.
4. Complete the review process within a 2-week period to minimize the potential for continued student failure.

After the referral is reviewed, a meeting should be arranged between the student, his or her parent or guardian, and the high school BEP coordinator. It is developmentally appropriate to solicit student feedback on the behaviors they perceive as obstacles to academic success. It is important for high school students to be part of the decision-making process. Soliciting student and parental or guardian commitment to the high school BEP program is strongly recommended. (A sample high school BEP referral form is included in Appendix H.1.)

Social and Academic Support: Combined Intervention

The combination of academic and social supports is critical for high school students demonstrating Tier II problem behaviors. Social support increases structure and opportunities for earning reinforcement across the school day. Academic support reduces the difficulty of academic tasks, which results in increased levels of academic success. The following sections outline the social and academic support cycles of the high school BEP. The academic support class provides instruction in organizational and study skills. The social support cycle, checking in, and checking out are embedded into the daily operations of the academic support class. In this way, the high school BEP effectively addresses academic difficulties and problem behaviors at the same time.

Facilitating cohesive supports requires coordinating efforts from a dedicated faculty or staff member. The BEP coordinator in high schools (1) coordinates the everyday operations of the BEP that are hallmarks of the elementary and middle school versions (e.g., screening, data management, student orientation, morning check-ins) and (2) teaches an academic support class. *Merging the academic and social supports into one class requires that a single person oversees the high school BEP.*

It is important to remember, that at the high school level, the BEP is not a singular social support but a cohesive academic and social support class. As an illustration of the importance of the BEP coordinator also teaching the academic support class, consider that a student checks in with Mr. Smith, the BEP coordinator, at the beginning of the day. The student shares that she needs to complete math homework before last period. If Mr. Smith also teaches the academic support class, he now has information that will guide the support he provides her during academic support class: he can prompt the student to complete her math homework and provide specific assistance in the completion of that homework. If Mr. Smith is not teaching the academic support class the unfinished math homework may well go unfinished and the student remains unprepared for class.

The BEP coordinator for high school must be a certified teacher. High school students should receive credit for participating in the academic support class. The BEP coordinator can be a special education teacher or a content specialist who has knowledge of and expertise in supporting students' academic and social successes. Depending on the level of need at a particular school, the academic support teacher can teach multiple sections of the academic support class. The academic support teacher may also teach basic reading, math, or other subject matter during the class periods in which he or she is not teaching or working on coordinator's tasks for the BEP. The academic support teacher may also have other behavior support responsibilities within the high school.

It is important to note that the role of academic support teacher requires active teaching, frequent interactions with students, and data management. The academic support teacher's role differs from other "mentor" models such as Check and Connect (Sinclair, Christenson, Lehr, & Anderson, 2003) in the following ways:

- The academic support teacher is employed by the school.
- The academic support teacher checks in more frequently (every morning and afternoon) with students.
- Students receive academic credit for participation.
- The academic support teacher is providing instruction to a small group(s).
- The academic support teacher may teach additional courses at the high school.
- The academic support teacher has basic knowledge of grade-level curricular requirements.

The following are critical organizational features of the high school BEP:

- Academic support/BEP coordinator

  - Dedicated hours for instruction of the academic support class
  - Protected preparation time for communication with general content teachers

- Minimum 45-minute daily instructional period
- Scheduled as the first class students have each day
- Low teacher-to-student ratio of 10:1, or 12:1 maximum
- Curriculum alignment with general content classrooms; for example, academic support activities would focus on test taking and study skills prior to schoolwide midterms
- Weekly and daily class agendas posted in the classroom
- A daily protocol that incorporates check-ins and goal setting
- Data reviewed and updated every 24–48 hours by high school BEP coordinator
- Twice-monthly review of student progress data by behavior support team

Social Support: BEP DPR Cycle

The social support cycle of the high school BEP increases structure, promotes contingent adult feedback, and teaches students how to ask for assistance within the school setting. The social support cycle consists of the familiar BEP features: morning check-in, feedback at the end of each period, afternoon check-out, and feedback from home. The important differences for high school are (1) added emphasis on student involvement in the management of the BEP, (2) the flexibility of the home component, and (3) the social support cycle takes place in the contexts of the academic support class (see Figure 9.2). The features of the social support cycle are presented here in detail.

MORNING CHECK-IN

For the high school BEP, the morning check-in takes place during the first 5–7 minutes of the academic support class. The morning check-in is part of the classroom entry routine that also includes:

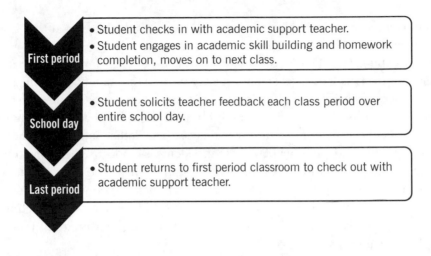

FIGURE 9.2. Social and academic support cycle of the high school BEP.

1. Daily agenda posted on the board.
2. Brief, 5- to 7-minute daily entry task designed to orient students to social and/or academic goals and morning check-in.
3. Brief, 1- to 2-minute daily planner check.

Organizing social support within the academic support class provides (1) an effective model of self-management and (2) practice in developing self-management skills. Students are engaged in self-management activities (e.g., planner updates, notebook organization, graduation requirement review) while the teacher models the self-management process to individual students during check-ins: How are you today? How is the homework coming along? I see you have a test coming up in history, how prepared are you feeling?

Many high schools provide students with planners or agendas. Systematically incorporating school planners into the academic support class increases student opportunities for self-management. Daily agendas for the academic support class should be posted and include specific details for activity completion. Students copy relevant information from the daily agenda into their planners, such as upcoming homework completion sessions. (A sample daily agenda is included in Appendix H.2.)

Teaching and reinforcing students' use of the posted daily agenda is beneficial in several ways. First, the practice of using an advanced organizer to independently complete class work is a useful self-management skill for the school setting. Second, when students operate independently, it frees up teacher time for the brief morning check-ins. The first-period, classroom-entry routine should take enough time to allow the teacher to make a full circulation of the room, thereby checking in briefly with each student. This requires careful planning by the academic support teacher. He or she must know the students' independent instructional level. Knowledge of students' instructional level ensures that students can successfully complete the learning activities on their own. The daily entry task, as an example, is an orienting activity that provides independent practice of core study skills. More details about the daily entry task are provided in the Academic Support Cycle section below. Careful instructional planning, in addition to proactive classroom management strategies, increases the likelihood that students will successfully engage in self-managing activities.

A plan must be established for situations in which the teacher notices that a student is highly agitated or in crisis. The teacher must quickly assess if the student can manage classroom activities with modest supports, or if the student is in immediate need of more assistance. If the situation is at or near crisis level, the teacher must be able to quickly access additional adult support such as a school counselor or administrator: accessing another supportive adult allows for immediate crisis intervention without taking the academic support teacher away from instructional activities. The protocol for accessing outside support should be set up at the beginning of the semester in anticipation of student needs, and not be a "knee jerk" reaction to a given situation. Outside support should (1) be available within a few minutes of contacting the main office or nurse, (2) link the student with a supportive adult, and (3) ensure that any safety issues can be immediately addressed.

A well-defined plan for identifying and supporting students in crisis during the morning check-in is an important consideration in decreasing negative school experiences. Students who are not emotionally prepared to participate in the classroom setting should receive additional needs-based support. Only when students are prepared to positively participate in the rest of the school day should they be handed the DPR card, reinforced for their participation, and sent on to the next class.

FEEDBACK AT THE END OF EACH CLASS PERIOD

Once students move to their second class period, the high school BEP cycle closely mirrors the BEP for elementary or middle school. Students give the DPR to the teachers at the beginning of the class period and receive feedback based on classroom behavioral performance at the end of the class. An additional component of the high school BEP asks teachers to include academic "primers" during the class period. During the initial daily contact with the student, the classroom teacher should deliver:

- Verbal praise for being on time, handing in the DPR, or attending class:
  - "Glad to see you today, Donovan. Thanks for being on time."

- A brief update on the period's activities *or* the big ideas of the day's lesson:
  - "Today we will be taking a vocabulary quiz first. Then we'll be finishing yesterday's reading on the history of civil rights in the United States."
  - "The lesson for today is about photosynthesis. The big idea of the lesson is that plants use sunlight as energy to turn carbon dioxide and water into carbohydrates."

In the last 5 to 10 minutes of the class period, teachers wait for a natural break in classroom activity to complete the DPR. They provide (1) a numeric score for the period that rates the extent to which the student followed schoolwide expectations and (2) a brief, positive comment about the student's classroom performance. As with the DPR in the elementary grades, the positive comment reflects at least one contribution the student made to the class, such as "Nice reading today!" or "Thanks for being on time."

As students retrieve the DPR, teachers should reiterate the positive comment verbally. The positive verbal interaction at the beginning and end of the period "sandwiches" the student's classroom experience with positive adult comments that are contingent on school-appropriate behaviors.

CHECK-OUT

The 3–5 minute afternoon check-out provides (1) a final, positive, school-based adult interaction; (2) reinforcement for daily progress; and (3) a reminder to organize and plan for work completion at home or during the following day. The afternoon check-out is in the same location and with the same adult, the academic support teacher, as the morning check-in. Having assisted the student with class work or homework during the first period of the day, the academic support teacher is in a unique position to follow up on homework and class work already in progress. This is a critical difference in the application of the BEP at the high school level. This *last check with an adult who is knowledgeable about students' academic tasks in progress helps students focus on the specific behaviors that increase academic success.* The afternoon check-out provides a follow-up check on academic progress. This continuity of support is extremely relevant and important for students in the high school setting.

Several factors in the high school setting make it difficult for adults to follow up on students' academic progress outside of the immediate classroom setting. The large physical size of high school campuses, a large student population (e.g., 1,200–2,000 students, or more), block scheduling, after-school activities, and compartmentalized teaching teams (e.g., the math team or the literature team) all contribute to an environment in which students are operating nearly independently, whether or not they have the skills to effectively do so.

The academic support teacher's responsibility at the end of the day is to ensure that students participating in the high school BEP have the materials and information necessary to accurately complete homework outside of school. It is critical to end a student's school day with specific verbal feedback focused on his or her academic achievement.

HOME REVIEW

To increase structure and support outside of the school environment, the high school BEP includes a home component. A parent or guardian is asked to sign the DPR and include a positive, written comment. The home component provides a parent or guardian with frequent (daily) updates on his or her child's classroom behaviors. Allowing a space for parents to comment or ask questions increases the likelihood that relevant questions and/or information can be communicated to the academic support teacher in a timely manner. Daily scores allow parents to reinforce student efforts or provide additional supports for increasing positive school behaviors.

As with the parent signature component for the elementary or middle school BEP, the purpose of the high school home component is to augment positive reinforcement of student achievement and behavioral performance. *The home component should not result in punishment from an adult at home when daily goals are missed or a student has a challenging day.* We recommend that parents provide extra incentives (e.g., movie night, extra computer time, a friend over for dinner) when students meet their daily point goals. We strongly discourage the removal of privileges, or any other punishment, when students do not meet their daily point goals.

For students who do not feel as though they can reliably, or safely, solicit a parent signature, a supportive staff member in the school can provide the parent/guardian signature on their DPR. The staff member receives the same orientation that a family member receives, is responsible for signing the DPR, and is supportive of the student's efforts. When it is necessary, this modification is critical for extending the network of positive adults with whom the student can meaningfully and positively interact.

REWARDS

The rewards available to students on the high school BEP should be meaningful for a teenage student and reflect student interests. Enthusiastic and creative efforts should be employed to identify reinforcers that actively link students to school events or activities. Some examples of social rewards that fit the high school environment include:

- Snack or lunch with a favorite teacher
- "Office assistant" or "teacher assistant" status
- Free or reduced admission cost to a sporting event
- Free or reduced entrance cost to prom, homecoming, etc.
- Free cafeteria lunch
- Pizza party for the entire class

Peer acceptance is extremely important for high school students. With that in mind, extending rewards to include a peer or the entire class may be additionally motivating. Again, a meaningful rewards menu requires knowledge of an individual student's interests. An effective strategy for developing a rewards menu for high school students is to solicit student feedback on the types of rewards they find reinforcing. (A sample reinforcer assessment for high school is included in Appendix H.3.)

DATA COLLECTION AND ANALYSIS

Data management for the high school BEP includes tracking daily DPR points for progress monitoring and for consideration of whether adaptations are necessary. The School-Wide Information System, Check-In Check-Out component (SWIS-CICO) is an appropriate tool for summarizing DPR data. The various reports available as part of SWIS-CICO allow the teacher to analyze individual student's overall daily scores, most and least successful periods of the day, and patterns of incomplete card data. Other graphing programs are adequate for tracking and sharing DPR data. To ensure timely modifications and identification of "problem" class periods, the academic support teacher should enter and analyze the daily point totals every 1–2 school days. More information on the SWIS-CICO and other BEP graphing programs is presented in Chapter 7 for reference.

In addition to frequent teacher review of DPR data, the high school BEP intervention must include at least twice-monthly meetings to review each student's progress and to create action plans to address areas of need. The systematic review of student progress data provides more opportunities for building self-management skills. Students receive supported practice in identifying classes in which they participate less than optimally and in creating action plans for increasing positive engagement. The critical pieces of DPR data management are:

- Data are updated every 1–2 school days.
- Data are presented in a graph that is easily interpreted by the behavior team.
- Data are shown and discussed with individual students at least twice a month.
- Data, stripped of identifying information, are shared with school staff at least once a month.
- Data are used for decision making.

Academic Support Cycle

ORGANIZATION

The academic support class is designed to provide supports in the form of (1) instruction on basic study skills to become organized and efficient and (2) daily assistance in the application of these basic study skills and in homework completion. *The utility and relevance of basic study skills is an important detail of the high school BEP.* The academic support class teaches skills that have a direct and almost immediate impact on decreasing the difficulty of academic tasks. For example, receiving time and assistance to complete homework immediately increases the probability that the homework will be completed accurately and on time. Providing explicit instruction and practice in study strategies the week before midterm exams increases the likelihood that students will be prepared to take exams. It is not sufficient to simply teach the study skills. Alignment of the academic support class with general content curricula ensures that these learning activities will have immediate applicability.

To ensure curriculum alignment, frequent communication between the academic support teacher and content-area teachers is necessary. The academic support teacher does not need to know the intricate daily plans of each classroom. A general idea of upcoming projects, tests, or quizzes, and the frequency of homework, is sufficient information for the academic support teacher to plan relevant learning activities.

In order to ensure that students have adequate time to complete all the academic support classroom activities, the academic support teacher must firmly establish and reinforce students' adherence to a daily classroom protocol. The daily routine increases predictability and maximizes student engagement. The daily routine should include the following:

1. Daily agenda posted on the board.
2. Brief, 5- to 7-minute daily entry task designed to orient students to social and/or academic goals and morning check-in.
3. Brief, 1- to 2-minute daily planner check.
4. Teaching core academic skills, 35–40 minutes.

or

5. Homework completion session, 35–40 minutes: (a) one-on-one assistance as needed; (b) student group work.

This daily routine fits with the 45-minute duration of a typical high school class period. There are two basic "formulas" for the academic support class:

- *Classes that focus on teaching core academic skills* should include 10–15 minutes of introducing a new skill with the remaining 30 minutes allocated to supported practice of the skill.
- *Classes that are dedicated to homework completion* should include 5–7 minutes of activities that help the students organize or prioritize work completion with the remaining time spent on homework completion.

BUILDING STUDY SKILLS

The Strategic Instruction Model (SIM) from the University of Kansas Center for Research on Learning served as the basis for the development of the high school BEP core academic skills (*www.ku-crl.org*; see Table 9.1). The SIM Learning Strategies Curriculum provides numerous variations of organizational strategies. The skills included in the high school BEP curriculum are not intended to address specific academic deficits such as below-grade-level reading or math skills. Instead, the academic skills included in the high school BEP help to immediately reduce the difficulty of academic tasks by teaching students how to organize their time and efforts most efficiently.

The high school BEP study skills curriculum includes:

- Planner usage and maintenance
- Notebook organization
- Test taking and studying

  - Preparing in advance for tests
  - Creating a place and a routine that is conducive to studying

- Goal setting

  - Identifying problem academic and social behaviors
  - Creating action plans to increase appropriate behaviors

- Utilizing school-based technology

  - Accessing and saving work to school server
  - E-mailing teachers

- Tracking grade progress

  - Progress reports
  - Grade retrieval on school server/teacher websites
  - E-mailing teachers

- Graduation plan

  - Semester-by-semester credit/class plan

As previously discussed, the sequence of the curriculum is as important as the scope of the curriculum. The sequence of skills presented here is one example, tailored to the academic

TABLE 9.1. Example Scope and Sequence of the High School BEP Academic Support Class

Weeks	Introduce (demonstrate/model)	Review/practice (guided practice)	Maintain/checks (independent work)
1–2	• Class expectations • DPR • Planner/assignment sheet • Daily entry task • Graduation plan	*Each phase of teaching will be guided by student needs. Students should be at 95%+ before moving on to another task.*	
3–4	• Goal setting • Tracking progress: progress reports, grades, e-mailing teachers, action plans	• DPR • Planner • Entry task	
5–6	• Notebook organization	• Planner • Entry task • Goal setting • Tracking progress	• DPR • Planner/entry task
7–8	• Test prep/study strategies	• Notebook • Goal setting • Tracking progress	• DPR • Planner/entry task • Tracking progress
9–10	• Technology: e-mails, server, Internet etiquette, plagiarism	• Test prep • Study strategies • Notebook • Problem solving	• DPR • Planner/entry task • Goal setting • Tracking progress • Notebook
11–12		• Test prep • Technology • Problem solving	• DPR • Planner/entry task • Goal setting • Tracking progress • Notebook
13–14			• DPR • Planner/entry task • Goal setting • Tracking progress • Notebook • Technology
15–16			• DPR • Planner/entry task • Goal setting • Tracking progress • Notebook • Test prep • Technology
17–18			• DPR • Planner/entry task • Goal setting • Tracking progress • Notebook • Test prep • Technology

needs of a specific high school. The sequence should be similar for 9th and 10th graders who are "new" to the intervention, but may bear modification for students who have been on the BEP during previous school years. These students may simply need the structure of the class to be successful and not require a strict skill sequence. The sequence of the curriculum should be flexible enough to accommodate schoolwide academic activities such as midterms, grade-level projects, and individual student needs. For example, if student feedback or academic data reveal that students are consistently earning poor grades on tests, the teacher may introduce test-taking and study strategies earlier in the sequence of skills.

As discussed in the previous section on Social Support, each class period begins with an entry routine to orient the student to the academic tasks at hand. The daily entry task (DET) is a major component of the entry routine. The DET is a brief academic activity that students complete as soon as they enter the classroom. It functions as an advanced organizer for study skill building and review (see Figure 9.3). Through DETs, the academic support teacher is able to (1) preview skills, (2) prompt skill use, (3) provide constructive feedback, and (4) reinforce the critical components of study skills. DETs should take approximately 5–10 minutes to complete. The remainder of the period can be used for teaching core academic skills or homework completion.

If students are not meaningfully engaging in the academic content, they will not benefit from the academic support. Instruction in study skills should require students to interact with the content in multiple ways: verbally, in writing, creating a project with mixed media, or teaching their peers. For example, when learning how to use a planner, students could (1) write the critical steps of planner usage; (2) verbally share the steps with a peer; (3) make a poster on the critical steps of planner usage; or (4) write an e-mail to a teacher. Again, stress is placed on the importance of making learning activities relevant for high school-age students. Students who have a history of academic and social difficulties in the school setting require additional motivation to engage in school work. Including pop culture icons, incorporating alternative writing outlets such as blogs, referencing popular musicians or athletes, or otherwise including students' interests in learning activities is highly recommended for increasing student engagement.

EXAMPLE: INCREASING STUDENT ENGAGEMENT IN LEARNING ACTIVITIES

A teacher notices that students are not consistently using their planners to track homework. She knows that many of the students are interested in cars. To increase planner usage she creates "Pimp Your Planner Activity," named after the television show *Pimp My Ride* in which people's cars are transformed from ordinary to extraordinary by a team of automotive mechanics and artists. The activity entails students decorating their planners to reflect their unique talents and personal characteristics. The teacher is using her knowledge of student interests to support meaningful engagement in academic activities (Kea & Utley, 1998; Klump & McNeir, 2005).

CONSIDERING ACADEMIC NEEDS

Attention to students' academic needs is equally, or more, important as knowledge of students' interests outside of school. Knowledge of students' academic needs extends beyond grades and assignment completion to the active inclusion of student feedback on the academic component of the high school BEP. The academic support class curriculum must systematically request and

Sample A

Think about your classes and your upcoming assignments, then answer the questions:
1. What is going well?

2. What do you need to do in the following areas:
   a. Homework (including missed work)?

   b. Tests?

   c. Projects?

3. When are you going to do the above work?

Sample B

---

1. Make a list of your classes with your favorite/best classes at the BOTTOM of the list.
2. Put your least favorite/hardest class at the TOP of your list.
3. Use this list to prioritize your time in academic support class (**TOP** of the list gets priority)

_____ LEAST FAVORITE/HARDEST

_____

_____

_____

_____

_____

_____

_____ FAVORITE/BEST

Sample C

---

1. Make a list of three study strategies you can use for the upcoming midterm in Biology.
2. Write down why each of those strategies will work for you. What is it about you that makes them important and helps you be successful? For example: I will draw pictures of the concepts because I am a visual learner.
   1. _____
   2. _____
   3. _____

FIGURE 9.3. Sample daily entry tasks.

utilize student feedback and must also balance core skill acquisition with homework completion. In pilot studies of high school BEP interventions, students repeatedly requested more time for homework completion. Often, for a variety of reasons, students participating in the high school BEP are not able to complete homework at home. Some of them have home lives not conducive to work completion, or they work after school, or they simply feel as though they cannot complete the homework on their own. Not only does the academic support class provide them with the opportunity to complete homework but the class uses homework completion assistance as a "vehicle" to transfer self-management skills.

The completion of homework serves multiple purposes critical to the academic success of students who are struggling with classroom success. It also provides multiple opportunities for students to receive reinforcement for homework completion, a behavior that is critical to the successful completion of high school. Students may move from "at-risk" status to "successful" and require less time and effort from faculty and staff if they (1) receive effective instruction in study skills so they are able to complete academic tasks independently; (2) receive immediate reinforcement (in the academic support classroom); and (3) receive delayed reinforcement (through grades and feedback from other classroom teachers).

It is recommended that the first 4–6 weeks of the academic support class dedicate at least 3 days each week to teaching study skills. As students master the core organizational skills (planner use, DPR use, goal setting), the class shifts to a focus on assisting homework completion with brief, core skill review activities incorporated into a DET. *Students' progress on academic tasks as well as student feedback should dictate the number of core skill or homework completion days each week.* The following is an example of applying student progress data and student feedback to determine the academic focus for the week:

- Students have mastered goal setting. Tracking progress is the next core skill in the curriculum. However, the students have a large project coming up and they need additional homework completion days to finish the project.
- Midterm exams are in 2 weeks. Students indicate they would like more homework completion days to study.

For students who require additional modifications to the academic curriculum and/or social supports, the low student-to-teacher ratio is a critically important feature of the high school BEP. A low student-to-teacher ratio enables the academic support teacher to gain a deeper understanding of students' strengths, weaknesses, and interests, and plan instruction accordingly. It also contributes to positive teacher–student relationships, which are critical to students' school connection (Croninger & Lee, 2001). The small classroom setting permits the teacher to (1) check in with each student individually; (2) manage the integration of general content curriculum with individualized academic support; and (3) more readily identify "red flag" behaviors, such as suspected drug use, references to suicide, or worrisome behaviors that mark conditions such as depression or anxiety. The early recognition of high-risk behaviors translates into immediate assistance within the classroom and school setting, as well as more direct contact with parents, counselors, and administrators, as necessary, to provide appropriate supports.

DATA COLLECTION AND ANALYSIS

As with the general, content-driven classes, effective data management is essential for instructional decision making in the academic support class. Grades for initial skill mastery, as well as follow-up assessments in the form of DETs, are powerful tools for curriculum modification and supplementation. Students should receive grades for their work in the academic support class commensurate with content classroom grading policies (e.g., percentage correct, adherence to a grading rubric, etc.). Student performance on learning activities should guide instructional decisions. Progress data should be regularly shared with BEP students as a means of increasing practice in self-management activities. Students should know how they earn grades on learning

1. In pairs, students exchange planners and critically examine their partner's planners.

2. Things to look for:
   a. Homework, tests, projects written in on due dates.
   b. Homework days for academic support class are written in on appropriate days.
   c. Student schedule is completed with class names, rooms, teacher names, etc.

3. Use grading rubric to assign each other a "grade" for the planner.

For each planner element, circle the most appropriate rating—0, 1, or 2.

Planner element	Easy to find, clearly written	Can find with a little looking, readable	Can't find or can't read
Name on planner?	2	1	0
Homework assignments written down **on due date.**	2	1	0
Tests written down **on due date**.	2	1	0
Projects written down **on due date**.	2	1	0
Homework days in academic support class written in planner.	2	1	0
Student schedule completed for red days and blue days.	2	1	0

FIGURE 9.4. Sample planner swap activity and grading rubric.

activities within the classroom, and they should know how to effectively track this information.

Self-scoring grading rubrics for daily learning activities are powerful tools for increasing students' self-awareness and self-management skills. Explicit instruction on how to use rubrics is important to ensure that students appropriately use the rubric to guide work completion and self-assessment. An example of a planner assignment with accompanying grading rubric is presented in Figure 9.4. As with all learning activities, the grading rubrics should be written in language that is understandable to high-school age students. The immediate and long-term relevance of learning activities is an important motivating factor for students to fully participate in core skill building.

EVALUATION DATA FROM A HIGH SCHOOL IN THE PACIFIC NORTHWEST

Contextual Modifications and Implementation

The high school BEP was evaluated in a high school in the Pacific northwestern United States. The school serves approximately 1,300 students and has implemented School-Wide Positive Behavior Supports (SW-PBS) for the past 3 years. During the previous 2 years, the school implemented SW-PBS at the 80/80 criterion, as measured by the School-Wide Evaluation Tool (SET): that is, 80% implementation of the teaching expectations and 80% overall SET score (Horner et al., 2003). The SET measures implementation of seven core features: (1) expectations defined, (2) behavioral expectations taught, (3) ongoing system for rewarding behavioral expectations, (4) system for responding to behavioral violations, (5) monitoring and decision making, (6) management, and (7) district-level support. This level of implementation is correlated with a reduction in ODRs for elementary and middle schools. In seeking to address the Tier II behavioral needs of their student body, the administrative team solicited the assistance of a university-based positive behavior support (PBS) team to create and implement a Tier II intervention. The intervention initially targeted social supports only, in the form of a basic BEP, with minimal student success.

Almost uniformly, the students participating in the BEP earned 80% of their daily points for a period of 1–2 weeks. After the initial period of success the students quickly returned to experiencing social behavior problem within the classroom setting. Repeated attempts to increase motivation through more meaningful or more frequent rewards did not have an impact on student performance. Informal interviews with the students revealed that while they considered the positive adult interactions valuable, their continued academic failure had the most influence on their classroom behaviors. The requirement to participate in academic tasks that the students consider aversive or unpleasant was the primary reason they engaged in problem behaviors such as being off-task or disruptive.

The high school BEP modification, marrying social supports and academic supports, was developed and implemented. Students were identified for inclusion in the high school BEP by the PBS team. The team met several times to review grades, attendance records, and ODR data, as well as anecdotal information provided by classroom teachers. Following the December holiday break, eight students were enrolled in the high school BEP for the duration of the second half of the school year. One student dropped the class after 1 month. For the duration of the semester, the academic support teacher collected student progress data in the form of grades, points on DPR, ODR data, and absentee records.

For a variety of reasons, the academic support class operated under partial implementation. The class met for 45 minutes every *other* school day to accommodate the schoolwide block schedule. Due to the alternating-day schedule, students carried a 2-day DPR and checked in *every other* morning. The block schedule also proved an obstacle to scheduling a check-out period at the end of the day. As a result, the high school BEP pilot did not include an afternoon check-out. Instead, the morning check-in doubled as a check-out for the previous days' performance.

In addition to scheduling obstacles, administrative and organizational factors detracted from full implementation. The behavior support team was unable to adhere to a consistent meeting schedule to review student data. This left all modification decisions up to the academic support teacher. At the time of implementation, a protocol for soliciting parental/guardian participation was not yet established, and there was not an emphasis on securing student commitment for participation. Despite being in the initial stages of implementation, many critical classroom components were firmly established:

- The scope and sequence of skills was well organized and accommodated the general content-area curricula.
- The academic support teacher entered and reviewed student progress data every 24 to 48 hours.

- The academic support teacher utilized decision rules for grading and instructional decision making.
- The daily agenda was posted and included (1) DET, (2) planner check, and (3) homework sessions at a rate of at least two sessions per week once the initial core skill building was completed.
- The morning check-in was a consistent feature of the academic support class cycle.

Fidelity Evaluation

Implementation of program fidelity was evaluated over a 2-week period at the end of the 2007–2008 school year. The evaluation was based on documentation of the critical features of the high school BEP. The social and academic supports were evaluated separately to guide decision making for implementation. Tables 9.2 and 9.3 outline the critical features of the academic and social components of the high school BEP that should be assessed during a fidelity of implementation evaluation.

The evaluation showed that within the 2-week period:

- Just over half of the students met the criterion of completing morning check-in for 80% of the days.
- The overall percentage of classes for which students received a teacher rating on their DPR ranged from 17% to 93%, with a mean of 53%.
- Two out of seven students returned DPRs with home signatures and comments, and for those two students, there was a 60% completion rate for the home signature.
- The mean percentage of class ratings accompanied by written positive teacher comments was 80%, with a range of 50–100%.

TABLE 9.2. Critical Features of the Academic Support Component of the High School BEP

Skill set
- Academic skills defined for the semester.
- Schedule of instruction (scope and sequence) established.
- Student evaluation plan in place for each skill.
- Students set goals for academic support class.

Daily class cycle
- Planner check each day.
- Daily entry task assignment each day.
- At least two homework completion sessions per week.
- Daily agenda posted each day.

Administration and organization
- Academic support teacher allocated with dedicated hours.
- Screening process utilized.
- Behavior support team meets every 2 weeks.
- Behavior support team reviewed data within past 2 weeks.
- Academic support data updated within past 48 hours.

TABLE 9.3. Critical Features of the Social Support Cycle of the High School BEP

Daily BEP cycle
- Check-in completed 80% of opportunities for 2 weeks.
- Check-out completed 80% of opportunities for 2 weeks.
- Class check completed 80% of opportunities for 2 weeks.
- Home signature completed 80% of opportunities for 2 weeks.
- Positive teacher comment present for 80% of opportunities for 2 weeks.

Goals and rewards
- Goals defined for BEP.
- Rewards delivered contingent upon meeting goals.
- Student participation in goal setting.

Administration and organization
- Academic support teacher allocated with dedicated hours.
- Screening process utilized.
- Behavior support team meets every 2 weeks.
- Behavior support team reviewed data within past 2 weeks.
- DPR data updated within past 48 hours.

These findings resulted in questions about implementation feasibility. One obvious problem that may have impacted the social support cycle was the lack of a consistent reward system. Students set academic or social goals for specific classes, but the goals were not linked to school-wide expectations or the points on their DPR. In modifying the intervention to accommodate student needs, most rewards were dedicated to students returning their DPR card or for students soliciting ratings from all of their teachers.

Student Outcomes

The following sources were used to provide a description of student outcomes for those students participating in the high school BEP pilot: (1) ODR data, (2) report card grades, (3) absentee data, (4) DPR data, and (5) teacher and student interviews. The Academic Support teacher compiled the data during the second semester of the school year using SWIS-CICO, class and school records, and interviews with students and teachers.

The student outcome data were encouraging but not uniformly positive. The most compelling student outcomes were reflected in the ODR data and student and teacher interviews. All students receiving ODRs during the first semester experienced a decrease in the number of ODRs for the second semester. All but one of the students reduced the number of ODRs to zero during the second semester (see Table 9.4). In comparison to national ODR data from high schools implementing SW-PBS, students experiencing two or more ODRs during the school year typically have an increase in ODRs in October or November and a second surge during March or April (Flannery et al., in press).

There was no change in rates of attendance or skipped classes. There was a modest change in the number of classes of the students who were failing. That is, just under half (43%) of the students reduced the number of classes in which they were earning a failing grade by at least

TABLE 9.4. Office Discipline Referrals for First and Second Semesters for Students Participating in BEP Plus Academic Support

	Office discipline referrals		
Student	Semester 1	Semester 2	Change
1	3	0	−3
2	1	0	−1
3	3	1	−2
4	0	0	No change
5	3	0	−3
6	1	0	−3
7	0	0	No change
Average	1.57	0.14	−1.43 ODRs

one class. While the school records did not reflect overwhelmingly positive increases in student attendance, interviews revealed compelling student and teacher perceptions as to the utility and relevance of the high school BEP.

Students and three general education teachers were asked to provide their perceptions on the following questions on a scale of 1 to 5. The English teacher, history teacher, and academic support teacher were the teacher respondents for the BRP cohort. The English and history teacher were chosen due to the academic and social difficulties many of the BEP students were experiencing in both of these classrooms. The academic support teacher was chosen because she would have, by nature of the class content, observed students improve on homework completion rates and organizational skill building. Each of the three teachers responded specifically about each of the BRP students. A score of 1 indicated no change at all and 5 represented a complete turnaround in student behaviors:

- To what degree have you noticed:
  - An improvement in classroom behavior?
  - An improvement in organization?
  - An improvement in the percentage of assignments completed?
  - An improvement in the quality of those assignments?

- Level of risk for placement change without additional supports? (1 = no risk, 5 = high risk)

Students and teachers had remarkably high agreement for ratings on improvement in behavior, improvement in organization, and improvements in rate of assignment completion. Students and teachers had relatively low agreement for risk of placement change. Note that general teacher agreement was evaluated by averaging the three teacher scores for each of the questions. "Agreement" indicated agreement in *either* increases or lack of increases in appropriate classroom behaviors regarding organization, social behaviors, assignment completion, and risk of placement change. Of special consideration is that even though the BEP social cycle (checking in, class-by-class check, checking out, and home signature) had low fidelity, improvements in behavior were consistently rated at a 4 or 5 by students. Teacher agreement for improvements in behavior met or exceeded 70%. Other interview findings include the following:

- 87% (6/7) of students reported improvements in behavior.

  - 71% (5/7) general education teacher agreement with student perceptions for improvement in behavior.

- 87% of students reported improvements in organization.

  - 86% (6/7) general teacher education agreement with students for improvement in organization.

- 71% (5/7) of students reported improvements in percentage of assignments completed.

  - 100% general education teacher agreement with students for improvement in percentage of assignments.

- 29% (2/7) of students reported improvements in the quality of assignments.

  - 57% (4/7) general education teacher agreement with students for improvement in quality of assignments.

- 43% (3/7) of students reported placement change risk without academic support class.

  - 28% general teacher agreement with students for risk of placement change.
  - 100% of the teachers rated risk of placement change at a 4 or 5 for all students.

Anecdotal feedback from content-area teachers was positive. There was an overwhelming consensus among the content-area teachers that the high school BEP had "saved" several of the students from dropping out of school. Also promising were the results of a pre- and post-survey conducted by the academic support teacher. Among other questions, she asked students to identify at least one adult by whom they felt supported in the school setting. The presurvey was given the first week of academic support during the second semester of the school year. The presurvey showed that only two out of seven students were able to identify a supportive adult in the school setting. The postsurvey showed that six out of seven students were able to identify a supportive adult in the school setting.

Even with the modest level of implementation of the high school BEP, students showed increased levels of positive academic and social behaviors. Considerations that would strengthen implementation include:

1. Clear, documented screening process (i.e., identification of which students are appropriate for the high school BEP).
2. Clear rewards system (rewards created with student input).
3. Fading and follow-up support protocol.
4. Increased intensity: 45 minutes daily or 90 minutes every other day.
5. Implementation of the check-out component.
6. Parent/guardian involvement in the identification and orientation processes.

SUMMARY

The case example provides a glimpse of student successes supported by the high school BEP. There is still much work to be done in addressing Tier II problem behaviors in our high schools. It is not surprising that students' age and their educational environments shift focus from fostering both social and academic development to fixed attention on academic development.

Students on the cusp of academic success are in danger of academic failure, increased rates of negative social experiences, and ultimately dropping out. We must rethink our approach to providing cohesive supports for students at risk. The high school BEP combines social and academic supports and takes into account the interrelationship between problem behavior and academic success.

The BEP intervention is relevant for high schools. Adaptations are necessary to account for the developmental needs of high school students and the organizational needs of the high school setting. With adaptations, the BEP is feasible and relevant, and it can make a difference in the outcomes for students at risk. More experimentally rigorous research is needed to support the development of the BEP at the high school level.

ACKNOWLEDGMENT

Preparation of this chapter was supported in part by U.S. Department of Education Grant No. H326S980003. Opinions expressed herein do not necessarily reflect the policy of the Department of Education, and no official endorsement by the department should be inferred.

CHAPTER 10

Adapting the BEP
for Preschool Settings

SUSAN S. JOHNSTON and LEANNE S. HAWKEN

WHY CONSIDER
IMPLEMENTING THE BEP IN PRESCHOOL SETTINGS?

Problem behaviors are often listed as the number one concern of early childhood educators (Conroy, Davis, Fox, & Brown, 2002). Individuals who engage in problem behaviors are at increased risk for rejection by teachers and peers (Walker, Ramsey, & Gresham, 2003). Furthermore, analyses suggest that preschoolers who engage in problem behaviors do not outgrow these behaviors; many preschool-age children who engage in problem behaviors will continue to engage in problem behaviors in elementary school (Campbell, 1998).

Increased understanding of the potential influence of problem behaviors on a child and/or his or her environment has resulted in an interest in developing interventions to address problem behaviors during the early childhood years. In preschool settings, researchers have explored the impact of primary prevention efforts related to arranging the physical environment, modifying the instructional environment, and incorporating the use of visual supports (e.g., daily schedules, choice boards) on the prevention of problem behaviors in young children (e.g., Dodge & Colker, 2002; Lawry, Danko, & Strain, 1999). The impact of Tier III prevention efforts with young children who engage in problem behavior has also been examined (e.g., Fox, Dunlap, & Cushing, 2002). For children who engage in the most severe problem behavior, researchers recommend developing individualized interventions based on functional assessment data (Sugai & Horner, 2002a).

As discussed in previous chapters, Tier I interventions may not adequately address the needs of all children and Tier III interventions are time- and resource-intensive. This suggests

---

Susan S. Johnston, PhD, is an Associate Professor in the Department of Special Education at the University of Utah, Salt Lake City, Utah.

the need for Tier II interventions, such as the BEP. Given the different developmental needs of preschool-age children and the different environmental characteristics of the preschool classroom, the use of the BEP in preschool settings will require some modifications.

MODIFICATIONS OF THE BEP FOR PRESCHOOL SETTINGS

In this chapter, we define *preschool settings* as structured, educational, early childhood experiences prior to kindergarten. We do not include daycare environments in this definition. Many preschools serve children between the ages of 2 and 5. However, for the purposes of implementing the BEP, we recommend working with children who are 4 or 5 years old. Children who are only 2 or 3 are probably not developmentally ready or able to benefit from the BEP.

Unlike elementary school, preschool is not mandated for young children. In most states, parents must pay for preschool for typically developing children. Children who qualify for special education can be offered preschool as part of the services identified and provided in their IEP. In addition, some children qualify for early childhood services in preschool settings provided by Head Start due to a family income level that is below a criterion threshold.

There are important differences between preschool and other school settings and corresponding issues that impact modifications to the BEP for preschool environments. First, preschool settings are structured much differently than elementary, and secondary school settings. Children typically attend preschool for a much shorter time period, often for a half-day, in either the morning or the afternoon. Second, developmentally, preschool children are just beginning to learn the rules and social norms associated with participation in a structured educational environment. Third, because young children need more supervision, there is typically one teacher and one or more aides (depending on class size) versus one teacher per classroom. Thus, the adult-to-child ratio is smaller than in an elementary classroom. Fourth (and importantly, for BEP implementation), each individual child receives instruction, guidance, feedback, and correction from multiple adults throughout the day.

Given that preschool-age children are just beginning to learn behavioral norms, parents may feel that a child who is engaging in problem behavior simply needs more time to learn the rules. They may view an intervention such as the BEP as excessive or unwarranted. Each of the factors described above should be carefully considered when modifying the BEP to fit within a preschool setting.

There is generally a greater expectation for parental involvement in preschool than there is in the elementary or secondary grades, especially in settings that serve students with disabilities. Goals and objectives created for a student on an IEP (with a parent as an IEP team member) often extend beyond the preschool environment to home or community settings. Previous research has shown that in terms of implementing the BEP, fidelity of implementation is weakest for the parent involvement component (see Chapter 2 for a discussion). This is a critical concern for the preschool BEP as parental involvement is essential to achieving success in meeting the social and behavioral needs of young children.

Most research conducted on the BEP has examined effectiveness across elementary and middle school settings (see Chapter 2 for a summary of the BEP research). As of this date, no formal research studies have been published documenting the implementation of the BEP in preschools. However, based on our work across the country, a few schools have piloted and adapted the BEP for preschool settings. These schools anecdotally report positive outcomes related to implementing the BEP with young children. The recommendations in this chapter are based on the experiences of these preschools.

When modifying the BEP for preschool settings, a primary concern is understanding that the developmental level of the child must be considered, as must each of the other factors mentioned above.

Many of the key features of the BEP can be adapted to address the needs of children and teachers in preschool settings. Table 10.1 lists the key features of the BEP intervention and the suggested modifications for preschool settings. Key features of the basic BEP intervention include (1) implementation is schoolwide, (2) intervention is continuously available, (3) students receive the intervention quickly, (4) time has been allocated for a BEP coordinator to oversee the intervention, (5) student checks in daily, (6) students receive regular feedback on a DPR, (7) students check out at the end of the day, (8) BEP coordinator summarizes the data, and (9) there is a team in place that regularly reviews BEP data. The majority of the features would remain the same when implementing the BEP in preschool settings. However, modifications will be necessary to make the intervention more developmentally appropriate and to fit the structure of preschool settings.

Programwide versus Classwide Implementation

The BEP is implemented schoolwide in elementary and secondary settings. That is, all teachers and staff in the building agree to implement the program and support students who have been referred to the BEP. In the preschool setting, whether the BEP is implemented "schoolwide," that is, programwide, is dependent upon whether the preschool is part of a program that houses several 4- and 5-year-old classrooms or whether there is only one preschool classroom in the building. For example, there may be a Head Start program with multiple 4/5 classrooms in one building. In this case, it makes sense to implement a programwide BEP. In contrast, some schools house a single preschool classroom within an elementary school building, and so the BEP must be implemented at the classroom level only. In other cases, a program may have multiple preschool classrooms but the classrooms are not placed in close physical proximity within the building. In such a situation, the BEP could be implemented programwide but each classroom would have its own process for checking in and checking out.

Prior to BEP implementation, consider whether there is a unified administrative team that can support implementation. Elementary and secondary settings typically have a schoolwide team in charge of developing the BEP and examining data for decision making. In addition, an administrator on the team has the ability to allocate the necessary personnel and financial resources to support BEP implementation. If the BEP is to be successfully implemented programwide across several preschool classrooms, it will require administrative support.

There will also be a need for professional development related to implementing and supporting the BEP. For example, if a preschool program decides to implement the BEP, the staff will need ongoing training and coaching on how to implement the BEP, how to respond if the intervention is not working, and how to adapt the BEP for use with young children. This typically requires that an expert in behavior intervention be available to the preschool program. It is often not possible to have an expert in behavior intervention housed within the preschool setting. However, many preschool programs are able to tap district or state resources to access

TABLE 10.1. Key Features of the BEP and Possible Modification for Preschool Settings

Key features of the BEP as implemented in elementary and middle school settings	Possible modifications for preschool settings
Implemented schoolwide.	The organizational structure (e.g., multiple preschool classrooms in the same district) and the physical location of the preschool classrooms (e.g., preschool classrooms are clustered together in the same building) will determine if the BEP is implemented classroom- or programwide.
Intervention is continuously available.	No modifications needed.
Students receive intervention quickly— usually within a week.	No modifications needed.
School has allocated 10–15 hours per week for BEP coordinator.	If intervention is implemented programwide, the preschool program will allocate 10–15 hours per week for a BEP coordinator. If the program is implemented classroomwide, the teacher or the teacher's aide will serve as the classroom's BEP coordinator.
Students check in each morning with BEP coordinator.	No modifications needed.
Students receive a copy of the DPR with schoolwide expectations listed and a numbered ranking system.	Students receive a copy of the DPR with classroom- or programwide expectations and a smiley face ranking system. An adult may be responsible for keeping the DPR.
Students receive feedback on behavior following each period or during natural transitions (e.g., 8:30 to A.M. recess) and receive four to six ratings per day.	Students receive feedback on behavior during scheduled transitions in the preschool classroom (e.g., group circle time to free choice centers, snack time to outdoor play) and receive four to six ratings per day.
Students check out with BEP coordinator.	No modifications needed.
Students receive verbal and tangible reinforcement for meeting daily point goal.	Reinforcement is tailored to the developmental needs and interests of a 4- or 5-year-old.
A copy of the DPR is sent home to parents for signature and return the following day.	No modifications needed.
BEP coordinator summarizes data for team meeting.	Teacher or aide may need to do this if not implemented programwide.
Behavior support team meets twice a month to review BEP data for decision making and progress monitoring.	Teacher, aide, and other personnel (e.g., speech–language therapist, special education teacher) meet twice a month to review BEP data for decision making and progress monitoring.

the necessary coaching and support. This is especially true of preschools that are linked to districtwide or statewide positive behavior support initiatives.

As with the staff in elementary and secondary settings, preschool staff should be given an overview of the purpose of the BEP and should be allowed to decide whether or not this program is appropriate and desirable for their setting. During the staff overview, questions will likely arise regarding the developmental appropriateness of this intervention for young children. Preschool staff may need access to research findings on the prevention of problem behavior and the effectiveness of continuous feedback and reinforcement.

Before implementation, the preschool classroom or program should have an effective Tier 1 prevention system firmly in place. Without good environmental arrangements and proactive classroom prevention strategies in place, the BEP will not be as successful for preschool children.

Overall, it is likely that fewer children will participate in the BEP intervention in preschool settings. At the elementary and middle school level, we have recommended that no teacher have more than two students on the BEP at one time. The same guideline should be followed in preschool settings. If, for example, there are three classrooms in a preschool program, the maximum number of students served by the BEP should be six. Contrast this with an elementary school with 12 classrooms for which there may be a total of 24 students who could receive the intervention.

The number of children who can participate on the BEP is further limited by the fact that preschool-age children are just beginning to learn many social and behavioral skills and require additional feedback and instruction to learn these skills. The preschool teacher and other staff (e.g., instructional aides) will need to provide more frequent prompts, redirections, and praise throughout the day to help the student be successful. In contrast, in elementary school, a teacher may provide a student on the BEP with feedback once per hour and consisting of a 1–2 minute discussion. If an elementary school student is struggling with a skill, the teacher can pull him or her aside toward the end of the day and talk about what needs to change, have the student practice doing the behavior the "right way," then provide a prompt for the appropriate behavior the following day. A preschool child, on the other hand, will need feedback more frequently, maybe every 20–30 minutes. A preschooler will also need to have the appropriate behavior modeled, with an immediate opportunity to role-play and practice the skill.

BEP Coordinator and Team

If the BEP is implemented programwide (e.g., across several Head Start classrooms within one building), a BEP coordinator can work with multiple children. If, however, there is only one preschool classroom, either the teacher or the classroom aide can serve as the check-in, check-out person. As mentioned previously, if the preschool classrooms are not in close proximity within a large building, there will need to be a check-in/check-out person (e.g., the teacher or an aide) for each classroom. This is due to the fact that preschoolers are too young to navigate independently through a school building. Since each classroom will only have two (or at most, three) children on the BEP, it may be more cost-effective for each classroom to have the aide or teacher serve as the check-in, check-out person, rather than to hire a part-time BEP coordinator.

As described in Table 10.1, another modification of the BEP for preschool settings relates to the composition of the behavior support team. Rather than having a team that reviews the BEP data twice-monthly, the teacher and the classroom aide, and perhaps a specialist (e.g., special education teacher or behavior specialist), examine the data to determine if modifications are necessary. If there is an administrator for the preschool program, he or she could also serve on the team that uses the BEP data for decision making. Someone on the team (or a resource available to the team) should have behavioral expertise and be able to provide support and recommendations to the preschool teachers and aides if the BEP is not working

Design of DPR

A key modification for preschool settings is the way that the DPR is structured. Multiple examples of DPRs for elementary and secondary settings were presented earlier in this book and in the Appendices. Figure 10.1 provides an example of how the DPR could be structured for preschool settings. Rather than listing schoolwide expectations on the DPR, the programwide or individual preschool classroom expectations should be listed. To provide additional support for preliterate, preschool-age children, it is helpful to include pictures that illustrate the expectations. Rather than using a numerical rating system such as 0, 1, 2, as is often used in elementary and secondary settings, a preschool DPR can utilize drawings of sad, neutral, or smiley faces to correspond to these rankings. Some preschools prefer to use a color-coding system such as green, yellow, red. One problem with this alternative is that a color-coded ranking system will increase duplication costs, as the DPR will need to be in color versus black and white. To decrease copying costs, the teacher could use a green, red, or yellow crayon to color in a black-and-white form to indicate how the child had done for that time period. In addition to the emotion face ranking system, the DPR in Figure 10.1 includes a model for the student to know what

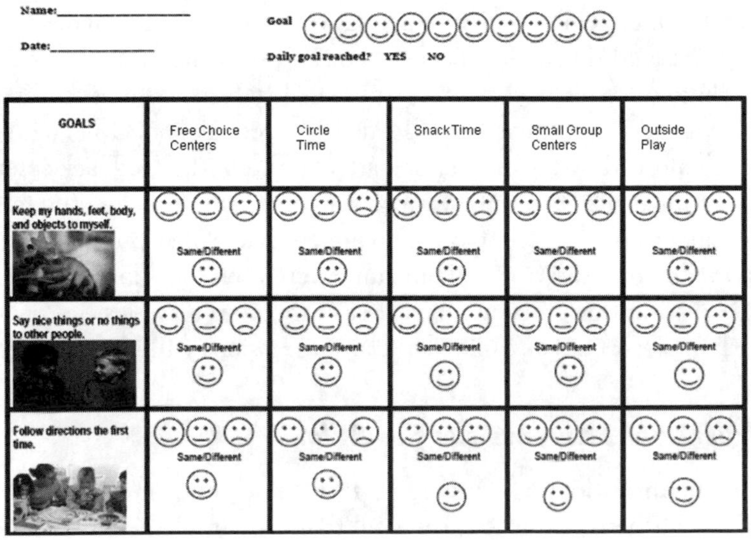

FIGURE 10.1. Example of a DPR for preschool.

ranking is desired. Preschool students are working on matching skills along with the concepts of same and different. There is a model of a smiley face so the teacher can ask if the rating that was given is the "same" or "different" from the smiley face model.

Across the top of the DPR you will see different times of the day that are specific to preschool settings (e.g., outside time, snack time). In terms of listing a goal for the student, rather than having a percentage-of-points goal as implemented in elementary and secondary settings, the number of smiley faces that the student must earn is listed across the top. In this example, there are a possible total of 15 opportunities to receive smiley faces and the student's goal is 10 smiley faces. This allows students to practice one-to-one correspondence counting skills, another skill that is important in preschool. At the end of the day, the student, with the support of the teacher or aide, counts up the number of smiley faces earned. Then he or she counts the number of smiley faces listed as the goal. At this point, concepts such as more or less are also introduced: "Did you earn more smiley faces than your goal?"

Feedback Sessions

As illustrated in Figure 10.1, preschoolers should receive regular feedback from a teacher or aide during natural transitions. However, preschool-age children will likely need more immediate feedback and redirection rather than waiting 30–45 minutes for the end of the rating period. Therefore, problem behavior should be redirected as soon as it occurs. Later, when it is time to rate the student's behavior, the teacher can remind the student of the correction that was needed. If the student requires redirection, a teacher will likely need to role-play ways to improve the problem behavior. In terms of teaching appropriate behavior, older students can be provided examples and nonexamples of the problem behavior and practice telling the difference between the two. In contrast, preschool-age children will need to have the teacher model the expected behavior and then have the student immediately engage in the appropriate behavior to demonstrate understanding of the expectation.

Preschool children typically enjoy interacting with adults and receiving one-on-one attention such as that provided during feedback sessions, even if the attention is in response to a negative event. Therefore, it is important for preschool staff to use a neutral facial expression and tone of voice when delivering corrective feedback or redirection. Otherwise, the child may inadvertently be reinforced by the one-on-one attention from the feedback session rather than understanding that his or her behavior was problematic. As with older students, preschoolers will need to be taught how to accept corrective feedback. Some preschoolers get extremely upset (e.g., drop to the ground crying and tantrumming) when they do not receive a smiley face on their DPR. To prevent this problem, preschoolers should receive lessons on accepting feedback prior to BEP implementation. Follow-up training sessions will likely be necessary.

Screening Preschool Students for the BEP

In addition to the modifications listed in Table 10.1, the manner in which children are identified for the BEP will be different in preschool than it is in elementary and secondary settings. As mentioned earlier in this book, students who qualify for the BEP in elementary and middle school settings are typically identified via some sort of documentation of their problem behavior (e.g., ODRs) or by using a schoolwide screening tool. If a preschool program does not collect systematic data on problem behavior, it may be necessary to rely on teacher or parent referral to select students for the BEP. As students are referred to the BEP, team members should discuss whether the problem behavior is a typical preschool behavior (e.g., difficulty taking turns) or if it is significantly discrepant from the behavior of same-age peers. The fact that a child is engaging in problem behavior does not necessarily indicate that the next step should be placement on the BEP intervention. The simplest, and first, intervention should be to assess what skills the child is lacking (e.g., transitioning from activity to activity) and to teach those missing skills, rather than starting the child on a more intensive, structured intervention.

CASE EXAMPLE

The following case example illustrates the use of the BEP in a preschool classroom. In this case example (see Figure 10.2), the key features of BEP implementation are discussed, with particular emphasis on modifications for preschool settings.

Ben is a 4-year-old with developmental delays who attends an inclusive preschool program for 3- and 4-year-old children five mornings per week. After his first 3 weeks of attendance, Ben's preschool teacher and classroom aide report that he seems to have more difficulty than his peers in adhering to the three classroom rules: (1) keep hands, feet, body, and objects to myself; (2) say nice things or no things to other people; and (3) follow directions the first time.

Ben's IEP team is comprised of his parents, his preschool teacher, the teaching assistant in his preschool classroom (Ms. Erin), an early childhood special education (ECSE) teacher, and a speech–language pathologist (SLP). The ECSE teacher and SLP provide services via weekly consultation with the other members of the team.

Observation of activities in the preschool classroom reveals that a primary-level prevention system is in place that includes good environmental arrangement as well as proactive classroom prevention strategies. Ben's ECSE teacher, who has extensive training and experience in positive behavioral support, suggested the use of a BEP for Ben and committed to providing ongoing training and support to the team throughout the implementation of the BEP. Initially, Ben's parents were reluctant about using the BEP with a child as young as Ben. However, after a discussion regarding the use of this intervention for young children, as well as a discussion of research related to the prevention of problem behavior and the effectiveness of critical elements of the BEP, all team members concurred with the ECSE teacher's recommendation.

There are 14 other children in Ben's preschool classroom. The classroom is located in the community center of the small, rural town where he lives. Because this is the only preschool program in this small town, the team decides that the BEP must be implemented at a classroom level.

Ms. Erin, the teaching assistant in Ben's classroom, will serve as BEP coordinator. Ms. Erin has attended a workshop on BEP implementation offered by the state office of education and has observed the implementation of the BEP in two other preschool classrooms in a neighboring town. Ms. Erin starts by collecting baseline data on Ben's adherence to classroom rules in order to obtain data regarding Ben's present level of performance.

The preschool teacher and Ms. Erin prepare for implementation of the BEP by creating and laminating copies of the DPR (see Figure 10.1) and placing the laminated copies in a folder

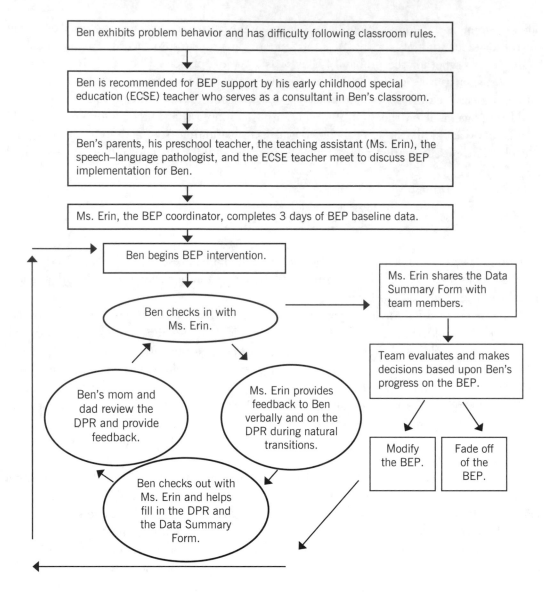

FIGURE 10.2. BEP cycle for Ben.

attached to the inside wall of Ben's cubby. Using a laminated copy of the DPR will increase the likelihood that the DPR will hold up to the "wear and tear" of a preschool classroom and allow it to be erased and reused. When Ben arrives at preschool, his mother prompts him to put his backpack and jacket in his cubby, take one copy of the DPR from the folder, and present it to Ms. Erin. Ms. Erin greets Ben and reinforces him for seeking her out. She also helps Ben to write his name and date on the DPR and discusses his daily goals. Ms. Erin demonstrates and provides examples of the goals that Ben is working on (e.g., keep hands, feet, body, and objects to myself) and talks to Ben about his goal (e.g., "What is your goal? That's right, it's 10 smiley faces!"). After Ben and Ms. Erin complete the check-in, Ms. Erin puts the copy of the DPR in the pocket of her classroom apron (so that it is readily available when she provides Ben with feedback during natural transitions) and prompts Ben to choose a center where he would like to begin his day.

Ms. Erin provides Ben with feedback and redirection immediately following occurrences of problem behavior (e.g., when Ben says something mean to a peer, Ms. Erin provides feedback on what she observed and she helps Ben practice saying something nice or saying nothing at all). Ms. Erin also provides Ben with immediate feedback when he follows the classroom rules (e.g., "I liked how you kept your hands to yourself during the story."). This is important because Ben's team recognizes that he needs immediate feedback regarding his behavior.

In addition to immediate feedback, Ben is also provided with feedback during natural transitions (e.g., free choice to circle time, circle time to snack time, snack time to small-group centers). Natural transitions in Ben's classroom are signaled by ringing a bell and rapidly turning the overhead lights on and off. Immediately following these transition signals (which occur five times each morning), Ben is prompted by an adult to walk over to Ms. Erin, who provides him with feedback on his behavior related to each goal during the previous activity. For each goal, Ms. Erin and Ben discuss whether his behavior is the same or different from the desired behavior, and Ms. Erin helps Ben to complete the relevant sections of the DPR by making an "X" on the face that represents Ben's behavior. (A sample of Ben's completed DPR is illustrated in Figure 10.3.) If Ben's behavior does not result in earning a smiley face, Ms. Erin talks with him about the reason why, and Ben practices how to meet the expectation during the next activity (e.g., "Let's practice keeping your hands to yourself at circle time."). This feedback takes only 1–2 minutes and is provided during each natural transition. On a few occasions, Ben argued with Ms. Erin about the rating that he was given. Ms. Erin has been trained to understand the importance of explaining her rating without engaging in discussions with Ben about whether or not a rating should be changed. Ms. Erin's rating is the final rating.

Immediately following the last transition signal of the day, Ben is prompted to seek out Ms. Erin, who helps him to count the number of smiley faces earned that day. In addition to being a

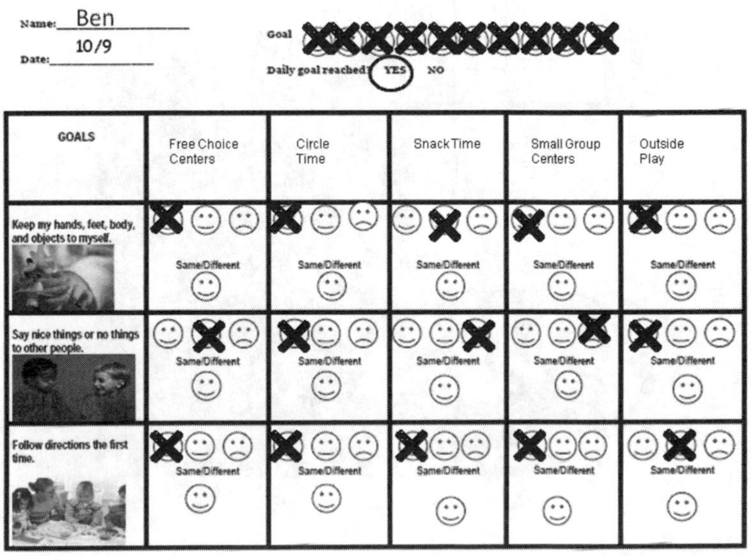

FIGURE 10.3. Example of a DPR for Ben.

critical feature of the BEP, this is a great opportunity to practice skills related to 1:1 correspondence and counting. After counting the number of smiley faces earned, Ms. Erin helps Ben to make an "X" over the total number of smiley faces earned that day, as well as to circle "Yes" or "No" after discussing whether or not Ben met his daily goal of 10 smiley faces. Then Ms. Erin helps Ben to graph his progress on the Data Summary Form (see Figure 10.4). Completing the Data Summary Form at the end of each day helps Ben to see his progress across time. It also ensures that the data is always up to date for team meetings (see below).

If Ben meets his daily goal of 10 smiley faces, he is provided with verbal praise, as well as a tangible reinforcer. Based upon interviews with Ben's parents to help identify effective, personalized reinforcers, his verbal reinforcement consists of Ms. Erin and Ben reciting Ben's favorite chant/cheer (saying "Super-Duper, Alley-Ooper" three times while swinging their arms in the air) and his tangible reinforcement consists of receiving a new sticker to put in his Sponge Bob Square Pants sticker book. If Ben does not meet his daily goal of 10 smiley faces, Ms. Erin briefly speaks with him about what he can do in order to meet his goal the next day.

As Ben checks out with Ms. Erin, she transfers the data to Ben's Data Summary Form and helps Ben to put the DPR in his backpack. Based on a discussion at a previous team meeting, Ben's parents know to talk with Ben about the information on the laminated DPR and return the DPR when they drop him off at preschool the following day.

During the first several days of BEP implementation, his preschool teacher noted that Ben needed reminders to check in with Ms. Erin at the beginning of the day, find Ms. Erin immediately following each transition signal (i.e., bell ringing and lights going on/off), and check out with Ms. Erin at the end of the day. However, after the first week of implementation, his teacher noted that he rarely needed reminders and that he seemed to enjoy participating in the BEP.

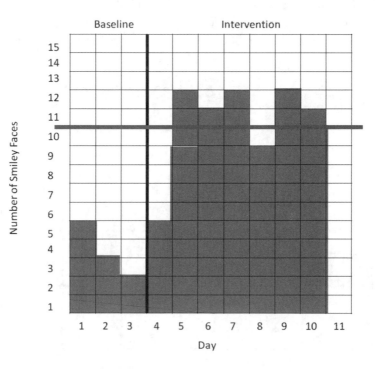

FIGURE 10.4. Progress Monitoring Form for Ben.

Using the Data Summary Form that is updated by Ben and Ms. Erin at the end of each day (refer to Figure 10.4), Ms. Erin is able to provide summary data for team meetings. Data for Ben indicates that he has met his daily goal on five of the seven occasions. Based on this, the team decides to continue with the implementation of the BEP as planned. Data is reviewed weekly during the regularly scheduled consultations between the preschool teacher, the teaching assistant, and the ECSE teacher. The BEP data is also reviewed monthly during the regularly scheduled consultations between Ben's parents, the preschool teacher, the teaching assistant, the SLP, and the ECSE teacher. During these meetings, the team discusses Ben's progress using the BEP, adjusts support as needed, and identifies ways to support the implementation of the BEP in Ben's classroom.

CHAPTER 11

Cultural Considerations
and Adaptations for the BEP

JOAN SCHUMANN and JASON J. BURROW-SÁNCHEZ

There is no doubt that the ethnic and racial demographics of America's school children are changing rapidly. In many schools, the student populations have changed so dramatically that school personnel struggle to find culturally appropriate ways to serve the needs of all their students. While the rapid infusion of diverse students can be challenging, cultural diversity can also be perceived as an important opportunity for school personnel to further expand their skills in an ever increasing multicultural world. School practitioners will approach this topic from differing viewpoints based on their education, training, and personal experience. For example, some school personnel may not have received diversity training in their formal education programs, whereas others may have received training from the school districts in which they work. Further, specific approaches to multicultural issues are influenced by one's own values, cultural background, and experiences.

In this chapter, we (Schumann and Burrow-Sánchez) present our view of the core components of cultural competence for school professionals, as well as provide specific strategies that can be used to culturally adapt the BEP to your school setting.

CORE COMPONENTS OF CULTURAL COMPETENCE

Developing cultural competence does not happen overnight or after attending a one-time training session. Rather, developing one's cultural competence involves a commitment by school personnel to be open to new experiences, self-examination, and exploring differing worldviews. Put another way, cultural competency is not an endpoint, but a lifelong learning process of

Joan Schumann, PhD, is a doctoral student in the Department of Special Education at the University of Utah, Salt Lake City, Utah.

Jason J. Burrow-Sánchez, PhD, is an Associate Professor in the Department of Educational Psychology at the University of Utah, Salt Lake City, Utah.

broadening the way in which one views him- or herself and others. Thus, we refrain from prescribing a specific set of strategies for one to develop cultural competency. Instead, we present general guidelines that offer flexibility that school personnel can adapt to fit their own place along this path. These guidelines are based on the work of Sue et al. (1998) and adapted for use with school personnel.

Knowing Your Cultural Background

School personnel are increasingly likely to work with students from diverse cultural backgrounds. Therefore, they need to have some understanding of how their own cultural background influences their interactions with students. In other words, we are all cultural beings and have specific values, beliefs, and biases that we carry with us and use as we interact with others in our world. For example, a school professional from a European American (i.e., Caucasian) background may hold cultural values such as rugged individualism (e.g., "You do things on your own"), pulling oneself up by one's own bootstraps (e.g., "If I did it, so can you" or "You just need to work harder"), strong adherence to timeliness (e.g., "There's no excuse for being late"), or high value placed on SES and possessions (e.g., "Living in a large home and earning a high salary is important"). Granted, the above cultural statements are generalizations about individuals from European Americans backgrounds. The important point here is that all people have values, beliefs, and biases that influence how they see the world, called a worldview. This worldview is based on a person's own cultural background. In fact, it is difficult to think of a situation involving human interaction that is not in some way influenced by one's cultural worldview.

We have heard some school professionals say things such as "I'm color-blind" or "Culture doesn't matter because I treat everyone the same." These types of statements are typically well intentioned, but also indicate a lack of awareness of how culture permeates our interactions with others. In addition, these well-intentioned school personnel sometimes do more harm than good because they may implement interventions with students that do not accommodate the student's cultural backgrounds. For example, a teacher may have read that when giving a reprimand to a student, it is necessary to obtain direct eye contact so as to further reinforce the delivery of the message. If the teacher were to assume that this behavior (i.e., direct eye contact) carries the same meaning across all cultural groups, he or she would be greatly mistaken. In fact, individuals from many cultures often find it more respectful to lower a gaze, especially when speaking with someone of greater authority. Being aware of your own worldview and how it influences your interactions with others is a good place to begin developing cultural competency. Such awareness will promote more culturally appropriate interactions with students from differing cultural backgrounds. Another component of developing cultural competency is having a solid understanding of the cultural backgrounds of the students in your school.

Knowing the Cultural Backgrounds of Your Students

We recommend that school personnel take time to learn about the cultures of the students in their schools, but we are the first to admit that it is unrealistic to know everything about all cultural groups. Therefore, we suggest that school personnel challenge themselves to learn about the values, beliefs, and practices of students in their schools who come from different cultures than their own. As one example, many schools we have worked in have student populations with a high percentage of Hispanic students. If this is true in your school, and you do not come from this cultural background, than it is important for you to learn about the Hispanic culture of your students. You are likely aware that the term "Hispanic" includes many subgroups such as Mexican, Puerto Rican, Cuban, and so forth. It is important to ask students what they prefer to be called. For example, some students may prefer "Latino" or "Chicano," whereas others may prefer "Hispanic." The same holds true for other groups: African Americans versus black Americans, Chinese versus Asian, and so forth. Your first task in this situation is to determine which of these subgroups your students come from and then make a commitment to learn more about their culture. You will likely enhance your work with students as you come to learn more things about their cultural background.

This type of *cultural learning* can include reading the professional literature and other relevant resources, participating in social events in the local Hispanic community and finding a culture coach. A *culture coach* is another adult who is familiar with the particular culture you want to learn more about and who can help in your learning process. It is ideal, though not necessary, to find a culture coach who shares your job title, as he or she will also understand cultural issues within the school context. In addition, if you are not familiar with the first language of your students, you can learn common, basic phrases in that language, to communicate more effectively with both students and parents. The ideas for cultural learning we described above should serve as a general framework from which you can expand, as well as apply to students from other cultural backgrounds.

Implementing Culturally Appropriate Interventions

A third area for developing your cultural competency involves becoming familiar with the most culturally appropriate interventions for the students in your school. Most of the school-based interventions for students with behavior problems are based on the values, beliefs, and biases of the mainstream European American culture. In other words, the cultural basis of many interventions may not be appropriate for use with students from a culturally different background. How many times have you heard a school professional say something such as "Wow, this is a great intervention! However, is it culturally appropriate for our students?" We imagine that you have heard the first statement many times but have rarely encountered anyone asking the follow-up question. Thus, a major goal of this chapter is to encourage school professionals to ask the follow-up question "Is this intervention culturally appropriate for our students?"

In order to address this issue we suggest that school personnel assess any intervention materials they plan to implement for cultural relevance for their students. Examination of intervention materials will be more effective if school professionals have already begun work on understanding their own cultural background and that of their students. We acknowledge that the developers of many intervention programs will not have considered cultural issues, so much of this task will be left up to school personnel. This is an opportunity to adapt the intervention materials to reflect the important cultural aspects of your students and school setting.

Cultural adaptation is the process of adjusting the delivery of an intervention to make it congruent with the cultural background of its intended consumers, without altering the underlying learning principles the intervention is intended to teach. In other words, cultural adaptation is the process of adjusting an intervention in culturally appropriate ways that will make its delivery more effective for the intended group of students.

We spend the remainder of this chapter discussing how these cultural competencies apply to the BEP intervention and the behavior support team. To further illustrate the process of applying principles of cultural competency, we use a case example of Ocean View Elementary, a fictitious school that represents a composite of several schools we have encountered. Our goal is to clearly demonstrate our suggestions and the lessons learned from working with schools like Ocean View during the implementation of the BEP.

Ocean View Elementary: An Introduction

Ocean View Elementary is a K–6 school with an energetic staff and a strong administration located in a diverse racial and ethnic community. Many of the teachers and staff live near the school and have made an effort to build strong relationships with the families and students at Ocean View. The cultural climate at this school is that of respect and appreciation for differences; that is to say, instead of viewing the language and cultural diversity as a burden, most staff members value the range of cultural representation.

Students at Ocean View come from all parts of the world and speak more than 30 different languages and dialects. In addition, most of these students are recent arrivals to the United States; approximately 57% are considered refugees. While many Ocean View families face the challenge of moving their family to a new country, several endure the additional process of healing from living in a war zone or escaping from their home countries. On the other hand, since many refugee families have been provided housing in the same neighborhood, they are able to use other families as a support system. They find Ocean View Elementary a great place to come together as a new community. At Ocean View, families feel as much a part of the school community as do the teachers, staff, and administrators. When parents are asked about factors that contribute to this welcoming and accepting environment, they comment on the interest that school staff show in learning about their experiences prior to coming to the United States. Families also cite how the school displays artwork and pictures from all over the world and that school signs are often posted in multiple languages, creating a sense of appreciation for diversity.

THE BEHAVIOR SUPPORT TEAM: ACKNOWLEDGING OUR CULTURAL REPRESENTATION

The development of cultural competencies can serve as a process for learning about your own cultural background as well as the cultural influence of others. We encourage you to consider infusing these principles while initiating the implementation of the BEP. While you may want to begin thinking almost immediately in terms of how the BEP can be modified to meet the cultural and linguistic needs of your students, we recommend that you also take time to reflect on the cultural makeup of your behavior support team and how your own cultural backgrounds impact your perceptions of yourself and others. For a list of reflection questions to help guide this process, refer to Table 11.1.

(text continues on page 168)

TABLE 11.1. Summary of Recommended Areas for BEP Modification

Intervention area	Cultural/religious considerations	Linguistic considerations	Socioeconomic considerations
Behavior support team makeup	• Do we have team members who come from a variety of cultural backgrounds? • Do we have team members who continually examine their own cultural bias and work to accept differences in all students? • Are we a representative group (e.g., in thought, experience, and background)?	• Do we have team members who speak another language? • Do we have team members who value accommodating for linguistic differences? • Are we a representative group (e.g., in thought, experience, and background)?	• Do we have team members who are familiar with issues of poverty? • Do we have team members who are familiar with community resources for families living in poverty (e.g., homeless shelters, food shelters)? • Are we a representative group (e.g., in thought, experience, and background)?
Referral system	• Is our referral system objective (and does our data reflect this)? • Are most students on the BEP students of color? • Are there some student groups (e.g., Asian Americans, Caucasian Americans) that are highly underrepresented in the BEP? • How can we ensure that *all* students at risk of developing more severe problem behavior are referred for the BEP? • Are our teachers using culturally relevant curriculum and/or behavior management procedures? • In general, do students of color feel a sense of respect at our school?	• Is our referral system objective (and does our data reflect this)? • In general, do students who speak another language feel a sense of respect at our school? • Do we have sufficient school staff personnel who speak a language other than English? • Do teachers view speaking other languages as a strength?	• Is our referral system objective (and does our data reflect this)? • Are most students on the BEP students living in poverty? • Are there different (or additional) resources that we can offer the families of these students, in place of, or in addition to the BEP?
School–home communication	• Have we asked families which mode of communication they prefer (e.g., written, in person)? • Do we spend time asking the family about their background and how the school can infuse their cultural values in everyday practices?	• Is there ongoing communication with families who speak another language? • Does our team have translators readily available? • Have we asked families which language they prefer? • Do we respond positively and quickly when asked to provide information in another language?	• Are we successful in communicating with families living in poverty? • Do we utilize several methods for communicating with families? • Are we utilizing an efficient method for noting changes in address? • Are we effective in providing additional resources to families quickly and respectfully (e.g., information about food/clothing/shelter, medical insurance programs)?

(cont.)

TABLE 11.1. *(cont.)*

Intervention area	Cultural/religious considerations	Linguistic considerations	Socioeconomic considerations
Reinforcement system	• Are the incentives we offer students culturally appropriate? • Have we asked families what they think? • Do we offer incentives that are not allowed in the home environment (e.g., edible reinforcers)? • Do we offer incentives which may be insulting to families from different cultural groups (e.g., books/games that perpetuate stereotypes of American Indians)?	• Have we asked families what they think of the incentives in their primary language (e.g., using a translator)?	• Does our student store offer meaningful reinforcers for students living in poverty? • Do we offer incentives that don't make sense for children living in poverty (e.g., video games when children don't have the technology to play them)?
BEP coordinator	• Does our BEP coordinator demonstrate cultural competency in everyday interactions with students and families?	• Does our BEP coordinator need to speak another language in order to communicate effectively with students? • Can we have a translator or multiple coordinators available to BEP students who speak other languages?	• Does our BEP coordinator understand issues of poverty? • Does our BEP coordinator have resources readily available to offer students and families?
Check-in and check-out	• How does our BEP coordinator respond when a child does not make eye contact, out of respect?	• How does our BEP coordinator respond when a child speaks in the child's primary language? • How does our BEP coordinator respond when a child communicates in English, yet with a strong accent, often making it difficult to understand?	• How does our BEP coordinator respond when a child comes to school late, hasn't eaten breakfast, or is wearing soiled clothing?

(cont.)

TABLE 11.1. *(cont.)*

Intervention area	Cultural/religious considerations	Linguistic considerations	Socioeconomic considerations
Data-based decision making	• Do our data show success rates across students from different cultural backgrounds? • Have we asked students and families what they think of the BEP?	• Do our data show success rates across students with different language types/levels? • Have we asked students and families what they think of the BEP?	• Do our data show success rates across students from different SES levels? • Have we asked students and families what they think of the BEP?
Behavior expectations and teacher feedback	• Do we have schoolwide and/or classroom expectations that may be culturally inappropriate (e.g., make direct eye contact when adults are speaking, participate in class by sharing comments frequently)?	• Do we have schoolwide and/or classroom expectations that may be culturally inappropriate (e.g., speak in English only)?	• Do we have schoolwide and/or classroom expectations that may be inappropriate (e.g., every parent must contribute $15 for the class party fund; every family must list an e-mail address)?
Troubleshooting	• Do we have parents and community members that serve as culture coaches for our teams? • Do we utilize these resources when our team encounters problems related to cultural differences?	• Do we have parents and community members who serve as culture coaches for our teams? • Do we utilize these resources when our team encounters problems related to cultural differences?	• Do we have parents and community members that serve as culture coaches for our teams? • Do we utilize these resources when our team encounters problems related to cultural differences?

What Are My Values?

First, as a way of defining *values*, think about the beliefs and behaviors about which you feel strongly. Consider the following questions: What do I think is important in life? What activities and actions do I prioritize in my life? Some of your answers to the preceding questions may have included things such as eating organic food, owning your own home, being married, making money, having new clothes, working long hours, going to church on Sunday, or being on time, among others. At this point, you may also recognize how values can vary greatly among a large sample of people. How does it make you feel when you think about people who have differing values than yourself? For example, if you prioritize "being on time," how do you view people who don't share this value? And do you think it makes sense for everyone to share this value? Why or why not? Continuing with this example, imagine what it would be like if the society you were living in valued time differently from you?

Where Do My Values Come From?

After you've identified what you find important and how your belief structures may influence your behavior and attitudes toward others, you may consider thinking about the origin of these values. For many, this may be a new idea, while others might be very familiar with how their values have come directly from their families or cultural heritage. Since much of this conversation is a personal dialogue to have with yourself, and perhaps your family and friends, we refer you to Figure 11.1 for a listing of additional reflection questions. As a final note, we remind you that developing your cultural competency is a lifelong process. We continue to learn about ourselves and others every day.

Ocean View Elementary: Knowing Their Cultural Background

When the behavior support team was first starting to plan for BEP implementation, they spent some time considering the cultural makeup of their team members. Specifically, they considered their own cultural backgrounds (language skills, native countries, socioeconomic status [SES], religious differences, etc.) and acknowledged that, although they had members

Knowing about Your Own Cultural Background
✓ What are my values? What beliefs and behaviors do I find important in life? How do I judge myself based on these values?
✓ Where do my values come from? Where did my family come from? How are my values similar and/or different from my family's values?
✓ How do I view people who don't seem to share these same values?
✓ How do my beliefs come across in the way that I treat others?
✓ Do I think it is important that everyone share my values? Why or why not?
✓ How can I be more accepting of others' values?

Knowing about Your Students' Cultural Background
✓ Do I know the cultural background of my students?
✓ Do I know which country/region/religion my students come from?
✓ Do I know if my students speak languages other than English?
✓ How well do I know the families of my students?
✓ Am I familiar with the strengths/challenges the families experience daily?
✓ Have I considered how to integrate my students' background into the daily curriculum and/or instruction?
✓ How do I make students with cultural and language differences feel welcome and accepted in the classroom?
✓ Do I have effective means for communicating with all families?
✓ How can I be more successful at building relationships with families and students?

Knowing about Culturally Appropriate Interventions
✓ Do we have a representative team responsible for implementing the intervention?
✓ Do we have an objective process for identifying students for the intervention?
✓ Have we asked family members from a variety of backgrounds how they view the intervention?
✓ Have we asked students from a variety of backgrounds how they view the intervention?
✓ Do the student interactions convey awareness and acceptance of differences?
✓ Do we have a data system that provides us with disaggregated data?
✓ Is this intervention working across a variety of student populations?
✓ Does this intervention provide for flexibility based on student, family, and community differences?

FIGURE 11.1. Cultural competency checklist.

from different cultural backgrounds, no one on the team was familiar with the refugee experience. Additionally, they quickly admitted that their perceptions of refugee students were often viewed through the lens of someone who has not lived the experience of being a refugee. One team member even shared some of the lessons she learned from having her values conflict with the cultural values of her refugee families. For example, this teacher highly valued sensory play with young children. She had also considered using items from a child's home to be a positive practice. With that, she often had dried rice and beans at the sensory table and quickly learned this was a problem for some families. Specifically, many of her refugee families considered playing with food, dried or not, to be inappropriate since in their native land food is often scarce. After sharing similar stories, the team identified the need to recruit some parents from the refugee community to join as a member of the team. By adding a "culture coach" the team would increase their knowledge base in regards to learning and understanding the cultural backgrounds of their students.

THE BEHAVIOR SUPPORT TEAM: UNDERSTANDING THE CULTURAL BACKGROUNDS OF OUR STUDENTS

Now that have you spent some time thinking about your own cultural background and influences, we encourage you to participate in some reflection that will help you in assessing your familiarity with the cultural background of your students. Before we begin, we must address a lingering concern that many teachers encounter, especially those who work in schools like Ocean View, with an abundance of language and cultural diversity. A common response we hear from teachers is this: "If I were to spend time getting to know something about every student's cultural background, I would have no time to plan my teaching!" We would like to validate this concern by saying we understand teachers' time is very limited, and often overburdened, especially for those teachers that volunteer for extra responsibilities (e.g., being on a behavior support team). However, we would like to offer a few examples of how teachers could allocate their time, take advantage of available opportunities, and in the end, save time and energy by making lessons more relevant for students.

Example 1: Ms. Ramirez

Ms. Ramirez was hired for a new teaching position at a bilingual middle school where most of students identified themselves as Hispanic or Chicano/a. As a third-generation Mexican American, Ms. Ramirez was not raised speaking Spanish, nor did she have much knowledge of her grandparents' cultural history. For the most part, her parents encouraged her to become more "Americanized" because they feared she would experience racism in school (as they had) if she were to identify as Mexican.

The year that Ms. Ramirez was hired, she was enrolled in a master's program at a local university. As she perused the course offerings, she discovered she had some elective credits that could be taken in any department on campus. Although she had already learned some Spanish prior to securing her new teaching position, she was still eager to learn more about the Chicano/a movement so that she could better understand herself and her students. In the end, she took two courses in the Spanish department, in Chicano/a studies, which served as credits toward her master's, but more importantly, brought about insightful discussions with, and about, her Chicano/a students. Upon finishing her graduate degree, Ms. Ramirez pursued her interest in learning more about how to effectively connect with her students by attending professional conferences and local cultural events. Eventually, her principal sought her out as a resource and asked her to identify a consulting group to provide ongoing professional development in the area of valuing and incorporating student cultural diversity.

Example 2: Mr. Farrer

Mr. Farrer had been teaching at Hoover Elementary for 18 years. Recently, he noticed how student demographics had changed dramatically. With changes in real estate and the housing market, many upper-middle-class families that once lived in the school zone had moved out of the area, and several apartment complexes had been built to accommodate families with low incomes. For the past 10 years, Mr. Farrer had volunteered at a church in a more affluent neighborhood. In the previous year, one of his students was living in the nearby homeless shelter. This inspired him to stop by one day and visit the facilities. Upon his visit, he realized how much help was needed to run and maintain the facility. Since he did not have a lot of additional time, he decided to change his place of service, from the church in the affluent community, to the homeless shelter where some of the students from his school stayed periodically. Now he feels he has a better understanding of why his students are often uncomfortable in his class. Mr. Farrer now views his curriculum, especially the examples he uses in class, through the eyes of children living in poverty.

Example 3: Mrs. Wong

Mrs. Wong is a special education teacher in a preschool setting in a rural community. As part of her job description, she is required to conduct home visits at the beginning of the year with each family. Upon visiting a home for the first time, she has found it helpful to spend time asking the family about their background and what is most important for them. She has learned a lot from listening to families talk about how they view their child's disability and how the rest of the family supports the child. Over the years, she has learned that other cultures view disabilities very differently from how she was trained to view them in her teacher preparation program. For example, she was taught to decrease atypical behaviors (e.g., hand flapping). Yet some families appreciate this behavior because they may simply view the behavior as "how he shows us he's happy."

These examples are merely a sampling of what professionals can do to learn more about the students and families with whom they work. We encourage you to use these examples as a springboard for generating additional ideas that fit you and your school.

Ocean View Elementary: Knowing the Cultural Background of Their Students

With the addition of the team's culture coach, Abba, a refugee parent of a student from Sierra Leone, the team felt more comfortable addressing student needs that they may not have been familiar with prior to Abba joining the team. Abba was glad to address the team's questions related to her community. When she was unaware of what other parents and families thought, she would simply ask them later that evening when families would regularly gather in the yard of their apartment complex.

One particular meeting was especially insightful for the behavior support team. During a discussion of the Daily Progress Report, Abba brought up an observation she had noted among several refugee students. These students had reported that it bothered them when teachers didn't use their real names at school. Abba had observed several students had lost respect for their teachers because they had made "English names" for them after saying, in front of the class, that their names were "too hard to pronounce." As a result, these students were being teased frequently and thus acting out more in class to rebel against their peers and teachers.

After hearing of this, the behavior support team addressed the issue with faculty and the administrator dedicated some time during a faculty meeting to learn proper pronunciation of names. For the behavior support team, it was a lesson in learning that, while many team members felt they knew their students well, there were many issues of which they were simply unaware. Needless to say, they were especially thankful for having Abba as part of their team. The administrator encouraged other committees to follow their lead in actively recruiting parents and community members to school-based teams.

CULTURAL CONSIDERATIONS FOR BEP PREIMPLEMENTATION

Building on the previous discussions of considering your own cultural background as well as the cultural background of your students, we are ready to begin thinking about culturally appropriate interventions. While there are many aspects of the BEP and many decision-making opportunities to comment on here, we have selected the most important areas for cultural consideration. Further, we have divided these areas into two broad categories, based on preimplementation and implementation decisions. We also need to note that it is not too late to apply some of the considerations in the preimplementation section even if you have already started the BEP at your school. Finally, refer back to Table 11.1 for a summary of these considerations (and more).

The BEP Coordinator: Awareness of Cultural Competency?

Just as important as team members displaying awareness and value for developing cultural competency, the BEP coordinator plays an equally important role in the effectiveness of this intervention in terms of its cultural appropriateness. Again, while other chapters may provide you with a list of characteristics to look for in an effective BEP coordinator, we encourage you to add "*demonstrates awareness and knowledge of cultural competency*" to your list of qualifying attributes.

As a reminder, instead of viewing BEP coordinator candidates simply in terms of "*Are they a member of a diverse cultural group?*", we suggest that you consider the elements of cultural competency as previously discussed. For example, rather than emphasize the color of a person's skin or the pronunciation of his or her last name, we suggest you identify important attributes, perceptions, and understandings this person is able to demonstrate. Put another way, it is more important that the BEP coordinator regularly demonstrate a high level of cultural competency through his or her interactions with students and families, than that he or she belongs to a diverse cultural group. For example, you will want to focus on how often the candidate considers cultural differences when making comments or decisions about students. Refer to Figure 11.1 for a more detailed list of considerations you will want a BEP coordinator to embody.

The Referral Process

How Do We Choose Which Students Should Receive the BEP Intervention?

The referral system is an area that requires special attention, in regards to questions of cultural adaptation. In designing the referral process for a school, it is important to have a thorough understanding of one's own biases so that the impact of those biases can be minimized and objectivity in the referral process can be maximized. Students should be deemed appropriate candidates for the BEP based on their behavioral need and the likelihood that they will respond successfully to the intervention. They should not be placed on the BEP as a result of teacher biases in regard to aspects of their cultural background. While developing the BEP referral system, the behavior support team should consider their personal perceptions about students "at risk" (e.g., students who are tardy on average once a week) or what "acting out" looks like in the classroom (e.g., consistent trouble following one or more school rules).

How Can We Assess the Impact of Teacher Bias on Our BEP Referral Process?

First, examine your schoolwide data. Develop a clear picture of the demographics of your school to understand representation in terms of (1) cultural, (2) linguistic, (3) gender, (4) religious, (5) SES and any other variables that may be important for your school (e.g., refugee status). Compare your schoolwide data with your BEP roster. Assess if there is disproportionate racial/ethnic or class representation in terms of the percentage of students who receive ODRs or who are recommended to the Tier II intervention like the BEP. Overrepresentation of certain racial/ethnic, linguistic, or SES groups for student ODRs (e.g., 95% of students who receive more than two ODRs per year also qualify for free and reduced lunch while only 25% of your student population falls in this category) may be an indication that Tier I interventions are working more effectively for some groups of students than for others.

If you find racial/ethnic, linguistic, or class differences in student referrals to the BEP, consider taking a closer look at how students are being selected for this intervention, especially if these are not the same students who receive frequent referrals to the office. In such a case, consider providing additional staff training or supports in an effort to increase diversity awareness among these teachers.

Home–School Communication Component

One of the goals of the BEP is to increase home–school communication. In implementing the BEP, a behavior support team should ponder, "What is the true purpose of home–school communication?" The purpose is to make genuine connections with the families of students on the BEP in an effort to better support those students. Given this, the behavior support team should consider how to answer the following questions: What is the most effective way of communicating with this family? How well will they be able to read this consent for participation letter? How can I help to make paths of communication between home and school easier for this family? A first step toward finding these answers is to seek the information from the student's parents. Remember, since the objective of the home–school component is to effectively communicate with families, your goal will be met when you actually do so.

These initial interactions with families are opportunities to develop a positive working relationship. Since many families are only contacted when something negative has happened, the behavior support team has the opportunity to reverse that trend and touch base with families about a positive support system for their child.

The behavior support team must decide how to approach families when their child has been referred for the BEP. Consider the following variables: (1) the best mode of communication for each family (e.g., written, phone, or in person); (2) preferred language (e.g., Spanish, Vietnamese); and (3) language level (e.g., beginner, fluent). Related to the language level, it is important to know if the family is fluent in reading the language used for written communication. This may not be information that family members are comfortable disclosing. However, office staff are often aware of challenges in obtaining written documents such as registration forms from a family. Access to translators who are readily available to assist in communicating with families would be an invaluable resource for behavior support teams. Translation resources may be available to an individual school through the district office.

Reinforcement System: Is It Reinforcing for Students?

A critical component of the BEP is the reinforcement system, that is, the quality and quantity of reinforcers that are available to students who are participating in the intervention. In order to ensure that the reinforcers available to students are culturally appropriate, the behavior support team may consider discussing this issue with parents, students, or the culture coach. In one school, for example, we asked students what they would enjoy earning as reinforcement. Several students wanted to use the reinforcers as gifts for family members. So here is a case where, had we relied only on personal judgment, we would never have thought a hair band would be reinforcing to a young boy. However, these young boys enjoyed using their points to purchase hair bands and barrettes for their sisters and mothers.

If the behavior support team chooses to use edible reinforcers (either in the school store or as prizes), the team should identify different types of treats that students are accustomed to eating at home (e.g., chili-flavored mango lollipops). A member of the support team could conduct a simple Google search and also ask students to list their favorite candy or treat from their part of their world (incidentally, these treats can often be easily ordered and shipped online). Additional questions for consideration are listed below. (Refer back to Table 11.1 for a more complete listing.)

- Do we have students who would be motivated by earning prizes for their family members?
- Do we have students who would be motivated to earn basic school supplies (e.g., notepads, pencils, crayons)?

- What items do our students already have at home? What could they use?
- Are there food items that are prohibited in the child's home for religious or dietary reasons? Does the family agree with the food items we use as prizes?

Ocean View Elementary: BEP Preimplementation

As the behavior support team made the final decisions before implementing the BEP at Ocean View, the team felt confident they were on the right path to understanding how to best modify the BEP to meet the needs of their students. First, they spent considerable time selecting an appropriate BEP coordinator. After listing all the possible staff, faculty, and parent volunteers, they decided to ask Rachel. She knew several families at Ocean View through her work at the refugee assistance center in the community and also was employed by the school as a paraprofessional. As a Mexican immigrant herself, she related to students who were new to the country, spoke another language, and often experienced feelings of isolation. Rachel also had a very positive and caring attitude toward all children and was well respected by students, staff, and families.

Rachel helped the team select a wide range of reinforcers that were likely to motivate students from a variety of backgrounds. The team also identified several parent volunteers who could serve as translators for home–school communication when needed. The team began to consider the issue of communication a bit more, and came to the realization that the English-only parent letters were used out of convenience, rather than out of consideration of family variables. The team decided that when a student was referred to the BEP, the school counselor, along with a translator if needed, would visit the family at a place of their choosing to talk face-to-face with them about the intervention. This came from a direct suggestion from Abba who was told by many families that this would help ease concerns about the program and increase understanding of how families can support their child on the BEP.

CULTURAL CONSIDERATIONS FOR BEP IMPLEMENTATION

Check-In and Check-Out

Do Interactions with Students Convey Awareness and Acceptance of Differences?

When a chronic problem behavior is first encountered, we are often quick to judge, without understanding the whole picture. As an example, when a student frequently arrives 10 minutes late to school, a teacher, without having an awareness of contextual variables, may view the child as "lazy," or worse, assume "the family doesn't value school." However, if the teacher knew more about the family's personal situation, he or she might learn that their water gets turned off periodically because of trouble paying bills. As a result, the mother must drive to a friend's house so that her children can shower before arriving at school. This is an example in which the teacher, left without any other information, assumes the family "doesn't care about school," when, in fact, the family cares deeply about school, and is making extra efforts to ensure that their child arrives at school ready to begin. For this family, being showered and dressed in clean clothes demonstrates to teachers that their children take school seriously.

This is one of many common examples of cultural misunderstanding. It is important that the BEP coordinator, who is responsible for having the first interaction with the student each morning and the last interaction each day, makes the extra effort to seek out relevant information and avoid cultural misunderstandings. These interactions are, in a large part, one of the most important components of the BEP intervention. Yet the effectiveness of these interactions may be hampered in cases where the BEP coordinator and the students come from different cultural backgrounds.

We briefly provide some ideas for working with a BEP coordinator to address this concern. The following example scenarios could occur within the context of the check-in and check-out process. The student (1) comes late to school; (2) discloses personal information about a family fight; (3) shares that he or she has yet to eat breakfast; or (4) states that he or she is scared of going home. Each of these situations requires the BEP coordinator to demonstrate care and respect for the student and family. For example, a response that does *not* demonstrate awareness and acceptance of differences would be the following: "You need to tell your parents it's their responsibility to feed you breakfast before school. We won't have time to find something for you to eat because the bell is about to ring." A response that *does* demonstrate care and respect might take into account the family's severe financial challenges that have resulted in an inability to provide breakfast at home and an unreliable car for getting the student to school in plenty of time for free breakfast. A BEP coordinator who is aware of these challenges could have some breakfast food available in the check-in area and provide the student with a few extra minutes to get some nourishment.

If there seems to be some misunderstanding or absence of positive interactions with a student, an administrator or behavior support team member should talk with the BEP coordinator about more effective responses to such a student. The coordinator may be unaware of (1) how to best respond in these situations, (2) may not know what resources are available to the student (e.g., extra breakfast bars in the office), or (3) may be in need of modeling from another school staff member in order to understand how to respond appropriately.

How Much Time Are We Going to Allow for Check-In?

If you find that many of the students on the BEP are not coming to school on time, you may choose to have a behavior support team member talk with families about this. After taking into account any relevant information related to this problem, the behavior support team can work to find possible solutions such as providing extra incentives for students who arrive on time, allowing for a brief late period for check-in, or providing transportation for families in need of additional support. Depending on the nature of the issue, we encourage teams to think creatively and keep in mind the larger picture, that is, to provide a positive first morning experience for the student as opposed to a punishing scowl from teachers for being late.

Behavior Expectations and Teacher Feedback

Are the Schoolwide Expectations Aligned with Home Expectations?

Does the family allow play-fighting while the school does not? Are there words or phrases that are allowed at home and not at school? If so, the team may consider teaching the student differences in those expectations. Taking time to discuss the differences (especially with older students) may help students to understand and recognize the differences between home behavior and school behavior. For example, in the case of play-fighting, the BEP coordinator could remind the student each morning that when at school, hands and feet must be kept to self, while acknowledging that at home it might be different.

Are the Teachers Providing Positive and Corrective Feedback?

Sometimes, teacher feedback becomes more effective when it is delivered, positively, in the student's primary language. For example, if the teacher used the same language at school as that which the student hears at home (e.g., "Bien hecho" in place of "Good job") the student may feel more receptive to feedback and increase motivation and effort. Additionally, it is useful to observe teachers as they provide student feedback. Observation of teacher feedback can help identify instances in which teachers need to be shown how to demonstrate care and respect for student differences as reflected in everyday interactions.

Data-Based Decision Making: How Will We Know If It Is Culturally Appropriate?

There are several ways to use data to assess the cultural appropriateness of the BEP at your school. Begin by asking, *Are the cultural adaptations we have employed having a positive impact on student's BEP success?* The most important thing is to be asking this question in the first place. If, as a team, you can recognize how your own cultural background influences your decision making, you are headed in the right direction. We applaud you for making the effort to respond to cultural diversity within your school context and for taking extra precautions to ensure your data provides evidence of implementing a culturally appropriate intervention.

Previous chapters in this book explain in detail the various methods for monitoring student progress on the BEP and how to use data to make decisions. Here, we add to that discussion by suggesting you ask these additional questions:

Do We Have a Way of Disaggregating the Data?

By disaggregation, we refer to looking at ODRs, suspensions, and expulsions within the context of student demographics. Look for patterns in the data. For example, are Hispanic students more likely to be suspended than white students? If so, does this represent an accurate reflection of behavior, or does it reference a negative bias toward Hispanic students?

In reference to the schoolwide PBS model, it is equally important for you to analyze your data to note any trends such as (1) disproportionate movement to Tier II interventions; (2) disproportionate success rates on the BEP; (3) disproportionate movement to Tier III interventions; (4) disproportionate rates in classification of students with emotional behavior disorders; or (5) disproportionate rates in expulsion. Many of these questions cannot be addressed unless you have a data system that allows you to examine these variables. If data on these variables are available within your current system (e.g., SWIS), the following information will provide guidance on how to use these data to note trends. If, however, your current system does not allow for these types of analysis, we suggest you consider adopting a data system that includes this feature. Without a schoolwide disaggregated data system, the behavior support team, at the very least, should be able to determine whether there are disproportionate success rates on the BEP.

How Is the BEP Working (According to the Data)?

When looking across student demographics, ask this question: *Is the BEP just as likely to be successful regardless of student demographic variables (cultural background, language type or level, SES, etc.)?* When evaluating student progress, you need to think of cultural biases and influences that could be affecting level of progress. For example, have you considered whether or not the student's parents are able to read the DPR? Are illiteracy or low English language skills the reason that parents are not actively supporting their child on the BEP?

To illustrate how disproportionate success rates on the BEP would look, refer to Figure 11.2, which depicts a school's success rates of students on the BEP. The proportion of students who are successful on the BEP across cultural groups should be similar to the proportion of students in each cultural group within the school. (This should also be similar to the proportion of students on the BEP.) However, the data for this school demonstrate that the Hispanic students are not as likely to be successful on the BEP as Caucasian or African-American students. Although some students from each cultural group were successful, it is important to look at the percentage within each group. These data indicate that modifications to the BEP for the Hispanic students might be necessary. If this trend is not addressed, over time, it would lead to a behavior support system in which a student is more likely to be successful in the program if he or she belongs to one group and not another. The main point here is to emphasize the importance of the BEP working effectively for all students regardless of their racial/ethnic and/ or class backgrounds.

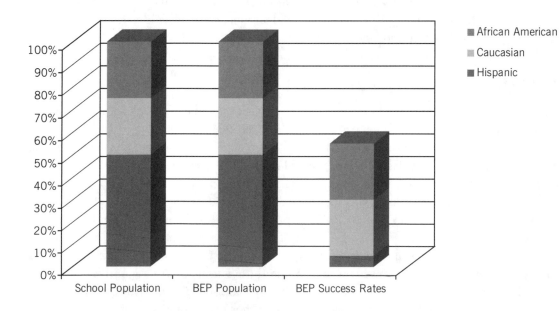

FIGURE 11.2. Data-based decision making to ensure cultural appropriateness.

How Is the BEP Working (According to Families)?

Have we asked family members how the BEP is working for their child? A second method for evaluating the success of your intervention across all student groups is to ask families about their satisfaction with the BEP. (See Chapter 7 for ways to assess parent and student acceptability of the BEP intervention.) In particular, talk with families of those children who are not responding well to the BEP. If you have spent sufficient time and effort in building relationships with these families, you may find they are willing and honest in providing feedback about the intervention. The family may not view it as their place to provide feedback to school staff, in which case you may consider having the culture coach on your team speak with family members about what is or is not working for them. Families who are less apt to talk directly with school staff may be more open to sharing feedback with a fellow community member. In either case, it would be especially important to respond with appreciation for any suggestions they may have and incorporate the feedback as quickly as possible.

How Is the BEP Working (According to Students)?

Have you noticed the students making comments about how the BEP is or is not working for them? For example, have you heard phrases like, "I wish there were Morinaga's milk caramel in the store" or "I hate it when Ms. Martin always calls me by the wrong name!" It is important to ask students directly how the BEP is working for them: *Are the reinforcers motivating? Is the teacher feedback helpful? Is the DPR understandable?* Especially when working with older students, asking the participants about the intervention is often an insightful activity for the behavior support team.

Troubleshooting

We know that you are likely to encounter scenarios of cultural misunderstanding that are not specifically addressed within this chapter. For these cases, we remind you to use your cultural coach, family and student input, and the team decision-making process to address additional needs and concerns as they arise.

Ocean View Elementary: BEP Implementation

After their first year with BEP implementation, the Ocean View behavior support team evaluated their data to note any trends among cultural groups. What they found was that, while successful among African American, Caucasian, and Hispanic students, they were still not achieving the success rates they wanted to see among their refugee students, especially those coming from Tonga. That year, they had four students from Tonga on the BEP and none of these students were having adequate success on the intervention.

After getting input from Rachel, they decided, as a team, that they needed to get more information from parents. They consulted a Tongan parent at Ocean View and she recommended bringing several families from the community together to brainstorm ideas. The team, eager to gain insight from the Tongan community, invited several families to the school for a conversation about how to best change the BEP to meet the needs of these students. In an effort to promote attendance at the meeting, the team also offered childcare, food, and beverages to families present at the meeting. The conversation proved to be a great success, with Rachel and the entire behavior support team present to hear suggestions for how to modify the intervention for Tongan students. The following year, the data among Tongan students greatly improved, with three out of four of those same students responding well to the BEP.

As problems arise, the behavior support team at Ocean View pays careful attention to any cultural misunderstandings that might be present before taking action. Parents and community members are frequently consulted to share insight and help the team troubleshoot various issues. In fact, at the end of each year, someone from the school asks them questions related to their satisfaction with the program. In turn, the parents feel an even stronger sense of belonging to the Ocean View community and continue to stay involved upon transferring to the nearby middle school.

CONCLUSION

In this chapter we have provided you with three core components of cultural competency as well as some concrete examples for BEP modification. Through the examination of your own cultural background and the cultural background of your students you will have a better understanding when trying to determine appropriate adaptations for the BEP. Keep in mind, when referring to "culture" we are using the term to apply not just to ethnic backgrounds but to racial, linguistic, economic, and religious backgrounds. Whichever stage of BEP implementation your school may currently find itself in, there are things you can do to appropriately respond to the needs and preferences of your students. Whether you are just getting started with BEP implementation or your school has had this intervention for some time, we applaud you for your efforts in thinking about how to modify the intervention so you can see consistent success across all students.

CHAPTER 12

Frequently Asked Questions and Troubleshooting the BEP Implementation

Implementing the BEP is relatively straightforward and takes a minimum amount of staff time. There are, however, common issues that have come up in schools that have implemented this program. The purpose of this chapter is to address frequently asked questions regarding establishing the BEP system of support.

WHAT IF A STUDENT DOES NOT CHECK IN IN THE MORNING?

One of the first questions schools ask is what to do if students are not checking in on a regular basis. Part of the duties of the BEP coordinator will be to determine if students on the BEP are absent or have merely forgotten to check in in the morning. If a student has simply forgotten to check in, the BEP coordinator delivers the DPR to the student and prompts him or her to try to remember to check in the next day. Although the BEP coordinator should not make a habit of delivering DPRs to students, if a student forgets to get the form, he or she should not miss out on opportunities for feedback and to meet his or her daily point goal. After all, this is a system to increase positive feedback and success of students at risk for severe problem behavior.

Other suggestions for students who do not check in include reteaching the check-in process (e.g., where to check in, what time to check in) and/or pairing the student with a "check-in buddy" who will help him or her remember to check in.

WHAT IF A STUDENT DOES NOT CHECK OUT IN THE AFTERNOON?

To begin with, the student receives a "0" if he or she does not check out. Recording multiple zeros in to the database allows team members to identify when check out is a problem. If students are allowed to bring their DPR back the next school day and receive points without having checked out the previous day, it will be unclear to the behavior team which students are checking out on a regular basis versus students who are not.

In terms of troubleshooting check-out, one of the first steps should be to ask the student why he or she is not checking out. Sometimes it is because he or she forgets and other times it is because there are bus/transportation issues. Many of these issues can be simply resolved by reminding the student that check-out is a necessary part of participation. Teachers can also play a role in reminding students to check out by prompting them toward the end of the school day (e.g., "Kiran, remember to check out when the bell rings."). This prompting from teachers should be faded over time so that students can become independent in participating in the program. For younger students, the prompting may need to occur for a longer period of time. We have found that placing sticky notes on the student's desk is another good way to prompt check-out.

HOW DO STUDENTS CHECK OUT AND STILL GET TO THE BUS ON TIME?

In some schools we have found that check-out is not possible after school due to bussing or other transportation issues (e.g., after-school care transportation). In these instances, when designing the BEP to fit your school, the last 10 to 15 minutes of the school day must be available to BEP students for check-out. You will need to get agreement from all the staff for this type of scheduling change. In addition, we have found that staff are concerned about students with behavior problems roaming the halls prior to the end of the school day. Students on the BEP can be given passes to leave class that are easily recognizable (e.g., a brightly colored, laminated pass that can be reused each day) by other staff who may encounter them in the hallways. Some elementary school settings have broken check-out into two short time periods at the end of the school day. The upper elementary (e.g., grades 3–6) students check out from 3:10 P.M. to 3:20 P.M., while the lower elementary (e.g., grades K–2) students check out from 3:20 P.M. to 3:30 P.M. This has led to fewer students roaming the halls before the end of the school day.

WHAT IF A STUDENT IS *CONSISTENTLY* NOT CHECKING IN OR CHECKING OUT?

The BEP coordinator should sit down with the student and determine what barriers are preventing him or her from checking in or out. For example, one student we worked with was not checking-out after school because he would miss his bus if he did. To resolve this issue the BEP coordinator spoke with his sixth-period teacher, and she agreed that the student could leave 5 minutes early from class to check out at the end of the day.

Some students may say, "I forgot to check in or check out." There are several solutions that can be tried. Enlist the help of the student's friends or siblings to remind him or her to check in and check out. Simple statements such as "Hey, can you do me a favor? Can you help your buddy Sean remember to check in in the mornings?" by the BEP coordinator often work. It is a good idea to reinforce the buddy you have enlisted for helping the student on the BEP. Another suggestion is to go to the student's last class and escort him or her to check-out for several days in a week to provide the student with practice with this behavior. Remember, some of the students are on the BEP due to poor organization skills and may need extra practice learning a new routine.

Some students may not check out because they have had a bad day and have not met their daily point goal. In these cases, there should be an incentive for checking out, even if the student has not met his or her goal. For example, the raffle system mentioned earlier, in which students received a BEP raffle ticket just for checking in or checking out, is effective. The raffle can be held once a week and only students on the BEP were eligible. The more times a student checked in and checked out, the more tickets he or she had, and thus the more chances to win. Raffle prizes were small and inexpensive, consisting mainly of small treats, pencils, or small toys.

When troubleshooting why students are not consistently checking in and out, it is important to determine whether the student has "bought in" to the program and is voluntarily participating. There have been times when a parent wants the student on the BEP but the student resists by not following through with the program requirements. Remember this is a voluntary, positive support system. Efforts should be made to find reinforcers that are meaningful for students who have not bought into the program. One student we worked with was having difficulty meeting the requirements of the BEP, but was interested in earning a baseball hat rather than receiving daily rewards. An individual contract was developed for this student so that after a certain number of weeks of meeting his goal he would be able to earn the hat. There will be times when students refuse to participate no matter what adaptations are made; for these students more individualized, intensive assessment and intervention are likely necessary.

The location of where students check in and check out is critical. It needs to be a place students can access easily, as well as one that is separated from the loud disruption of common areas such as hallways and cafeterias. In some schools where we have seen inconsistency in students checking in and out, either the location was inconvenient (i.e., not centrally located) or there had not been a permanent place set up for the process. For example, one of the schools we worked in chose the library as a check-in/check-out location. This location usually worked well, but was not available at times when parent groups met in the library after school, which disrupted the check-out process.

Although the check-in/check-out location needs to be in a quiet area, it does help if it is located near a common area so that the BEP coordinator can scan the area to look for students who have not checked in. It is important to build independence in the process of participating in the BEP, but it also helps to provide prompts to students who may need them. In middle schools, in particular, students are heavily invested in peer interaction. It may take some prompting to help break them away from their peers to check in.

WHAT IF *SEVERAL* STUDENTS ARE NOT CHECKING IN AND CHECKING OUT?

If several students are not checking in and out, the implementation of the whole intervention needs to be examined. One question that should be answered is *Has the school given the BEP a high profile?* Elsewhere in this book we describe how to give the BEP a high profile and ensure that it is a positive intervention. Without that boost, the BEP may be seen as just another educational innovation that will pass with time. In one of the schools we worked with, the staff were not well trained on how to implement the intervention. There was disagreement as to which students should be placed on the BEP, and issues were raised about existing programs that interfered or overlapped with the BEP. In that school, there were some staff who were "sabotaging" the intervention. That is, since the staff members were not in agreement with how the BEP should be implemented and with whom, they did not put much effort into the intervention and were not providing students with regular feedback. From this experience, we have learned that schools should complete the BEP Implementation Readiness Questionnaire. Staff commitment prior to implementation is critical to achieving success with this system of support.

Another question to consider is, *Is the BEP coordinator a person whom students enjoy and look forward to interacting with?* In some of the schools in which we have worked, the BEP coordinator is chosen based on time availability, rather than on his or her personality "fit" with the students. Although educators often go into the business of working in schools in part because they enjoy working with children, there are usually certain teachers or paraprofessionals that the students really resonate with, enjoy being around, and for whom they will work hard. In one of the middle schools we worked in, the BEP coordinator had an art of joking with students to improve their moods or reduce tension. These students could not wait to interact with her on a daily basis, and she was often sought out for problem solving with other staff around student issues.

In another school we worked in, the BEP coordinator was a paraprofessional who was placed in the position out of default: she was available before and after school. Although she was very effective in supporting teachers, she did not really want the job as BEP coordinator, and this came through in her interactions with students. She was often curt with them, more negative than positive, and had a hard time managing the numbers of students who were checking in and out daily. She would complain in front of students that she did not like the BEP. It is easy to see why, over time, students would not want to engage in the BEP intervention in this situation.

WHAT IF STUDENTS WHO DO NOT NEED THE BEP WANT TO BE ON IT IN ORDER TO EARN REINFORCERS AND RECEIVE ADULT ATTENTION?

Schools across the country have asked this question. We see this trend in elementary schools more often than in middle or high school settings. Younger students tend to seek out adult attention more than older students. As kids get older, peer attention becomes more important than adult attention.

In terms of solving this issue, several things can be done during the setup of the BEP to reduce the likelihood that it will become a problem. We often hear, from students and staff, that it is not "fair" for students with behavior problems to receive extra attention and reinforcement. First, staff members need to understand and believe that being "fair" does not mean doing the same thing with each student, but rather giving each student what he or she needs to be successful.

Oftentimes, staff members have a harder time accepting the extra attention received by the BEP students than do non-BEP students. Students are used to seeing other students pulled out for services (e.g., special education, speech and language therapy, counseling) and getting additional attention/instruction for their identified needs. The BEP is similar to these supplementary services in that we are providing services to students who need them, rather than providing a supplementary intervention to all students.

It is important to assess whether or not your schoolwide Tier I reinforcement system (e.g., schoolwide token system for following behavioral expectations) is working well and if students who are engaging in appropriate behavior the majority of the time are getting acknowledged consistently for their behavior. Some of the schools we work in keep track of the number of positives (i.e., tokens or tickets) that are given out by school personnel as a way to ensure that all students in the school are receiving reinforcement.

The next step is to ensure that check-in and check-out occurs in a nonpublic location so that the extra attention and reinforcement are not as salient to other students. We have found that if other students, particularly younger students, see the check-in and check-out process they are more likely to want to be involved. Students who are on the BEP should be taught not to flaunt and antagonize other children with the reinforcers that they have earned. For example, if students earn a tangible reinforcer (e.g., small toy), they should be taught to put it in their backpacks and not take it out until they are away from the other students in the school.

Another way to reduce the desire for students to be on the intervention is to limit the distribution of reinforcers that are tangible items, such as candy, food, and toys. The goal of the intervention is for students to receive more feedback and reinforcement for appropriate behavior. This reinforcement does not need to be in the form of something tangible. Having students earn activities and time with preferred adults or other peers will also help reduce the desire by other students to be on the intervention. In some of our schools, students who are on the BEP can earn reinforcers for their whole class, or can include four to five peers who are not on the intervention. Finally, if certain students are heavily invested in being on the BEP, perhaps they can serve as helpers during check-in and check-out. That way, they can receive the extra adult attention but also not have to engage in the full intervention.

SINCE THE BEP IS AN INTERVENTION FOR STUDENTS AT RISK, SHOULD STUDENTS ALREADY IDENTIFIED AS HAVING A DISABILITY BE INCLUDED IN THE INTERVENTION?

Yes, if they are also appropriate candidates for the BEP. The BEP is designed to support students who are at risk but are not currently engaging in severe problem behavior. Many students who have learning or communication disabilities may just be beginning to engage in problem behavior. These students are perfect candidates for the BEP, as the goal is to prevent students from entering a higher risk group. The main issue when assessing the appropriateness of students with disabilities for the BEP is to gather a quick assessment of the function of the student's problem behavior. Many students with learning disabilities may be acting out because the work is too difficult, so it is important to determine if the material is being taught at the student's instructional level.

Students with emotional and behavior disabilities likely require more intensive intervention than the BEP can provide. These students have individualized IEP goals for behavior. Since the BEP is administered similarly across students, it does not support the individualized requirement of the IEP. Students with more severe disabilities (e.g., serious cognitive delays) can benefit from the program, but may need additional support to successfully participate on the BEP. For more information about adapting the BEP for students with severe disabilities, see Hawken and O'Neill (2006).

HOW MANY STUDENTS CAN ONE BEP COORDINATOR SUPPORT? CAN THERE BE MORE THAN ONE BEP COORDINATOR?

Our experience tells us that for elementary school students, one BEP coordinator can support 15 to 20 students at a time. For middle and high school settings, up to 30 students can be supported by one BEP coordinator. The number of students that can be supported depends *greatly* on the skills of the BEP coordinator to manage groups of students. Some BEP coordinators become frazzled with too many students in a room, whereas others are comfortable checking in multiple students at a time. What has happened frequently in our schools is that students will need to be taught the check-in/check-out process as well as what to do when they are waiting to check in and out. One school we worked in had a line of tape on the floor to indicate where students were supposed to stand while waiting to check in or out.

An additional factor in determining how many students can be supported depends on whether check-in and check-out can occur at staggered times. For example, if the school allows check-in 20 to 30 minutes prior to school, this allows students to stagger the check-in process. If check-in is only 10 minutes prior to school, it will be more difficult to have as many students on the program.

We are often asked, *What if we have more than 30 students who need the BEP?* There are several answers to this question. First of all, the BEP should be only one type of Tier II intervention that is implemented in your school. There should be a menu of other Tier II interventions to support students who are at risk. If, however, the staff feel that more students can benefit from the intervention, it would be wise to have more than one BEP coordinator. We have also seen the need for more than one BEP coordinator if a school building is rather large or houses multiple floors. Some schools will have a BEP coordinator per wing of the school or per floor.

We have also been asked whether one person can do check-in, and a second person can lead check-out. As long as the assigned person is consistent across days (e.g., students check in with the Ms. Singh every morning and check out with Mr. Myer every afternoon) this tends to work fine. Also, it is critical that these two BEP coordinators communicate regularly about how the students are doing, and predetermine who will complete tasks such as entering data into the computer on a regular basis. It does not work if every day there are different people leading check-in/check-out, for example, if on Monday it is one staff member, on Tuesday a different person, and so on. One goal of the BEP is to build a positive connection with an adult. This is difficult to do if the adult is always changing from day to day.

WHAT IF THE STUDENT LOSES HIS OR HER DPR?

One of the responsibilities for the student on the BEP includes carrying the DPR from class to class, teacher to teacher, or, in the case of elementary school students, from setting to setting. We recommend teaching the students to get another DPR as soon as they realize they have lost it. That way, although they may have lost some points toward their goal by losing the DPR, they have not lost their points for the entire day. They can receive feedback on their new DPR and continue to receive positive feedback throughout the day. For younger students, some may need the DPR to be placed on a clipboard so that it is less likely to get lost during transitions. In some schools we have worked in, classroom teachers keep extra copies of the DPRs, in case a student loses one.

Students may also "lose" DPR cards if they find that being on the BEP is not helpful or rewarding. For such students, troubleshoot ways to improve the program. Often this involves asking the student what types of rewards they are interested in working for. Some students may "lose" their DPR if they have had a bad day and are afraid to bring the DPR home to their parents. As sad as it may be, there have been parents who punish students severely for having a "bad day" at school. In these situations, we have either encouraged the parents to use the program positively, or we have had students not take their cards home as part of the program. We cannot overemphasize that the BEP needs to be a positive program, one the students enjoy participating in. If the student gets into even more trouble by being on the BEP, he or she is going to be unlikely to participate.

WHAT HAPPENS WHEN A STUDENT GETS AN ODR IN AN UNSTRUCTURED SETTING AND IT IS NOT REFLECTED ON THE DPR?

The BEP targets student behavior in the classroom throughout the day. Often, however, students on the BEP receive a referral on the playground, in the hallway, or in the lunchroom, and this is not reflected on the DPR. On a few occasions, students get into a fight at recess, but do well enough in the classroom to earn enough points to get a reward at the end of the day. In such an instance, teachers become upset. They feel the student did not deserve to earn a reward because of the major infraction. Schools we have worked with have chosen different ways to address this issue. Some schools will deduct an automatic 20 points from the DPR for any ODR. This means that unless the student has had an otherwise perfect day, he or she is not likely to meet the daily point goal. Other schools do not want to institute a response cost (i.e., removal of points) for ODRs. Instead, these schools do not allow students to earn a reward on a day an ODR is obtained or to exchange points for a larger reward. Whatever system of consequences is put into place, there must be good communication between school staff and the BEP coordinator when students receive ODRs, so that this situation is always handled consistently.

HOW DO CHECK-IN AND CHECK-OUT OCCUR WITH MULTIPLE STUDENTS? HOW DOES EACH STUDENT GET ONE-ON-ONE ATTENTION?

The purpose of check-in and check-out is to provide a positive link to an adult other than the student's teacher. Check-in and check-out are not counseling sessions, but rather quick, positive, and brief interactions that provide students with prompts about things to work on. If a student is having a difficult time (e.g., just got into a fight or is crying), the BEP coordinator can ask the student to have a seat and spend more time with him or her after the check-in process is complete for all students. In some circumstances, it is more appropriate to ask for help from the counselor, school psychologist, or principal if the student is seriously distressed.

How well multiple students are handled at a time depends greatly on the skills of the BEP coordinator. All of the materials for the students and for the check-in and check-out process should be well organized and easily accessible to the BEP coordinator. In addition, many elements of check-in can be completed by the student. For example, students can write their own names on their DPRs each morning. During check-out, students can calculate their own percentage of points. Students on the BEP receive brief, one-on-one adult attention, not only in the morning and afternoon, but from their classroom teacher(s) throughout the day. Also, the BEP coordinator is typically a member of the school staff and therefore sees the students throughout the day to provide additional attention. For example, in some of our schools the BEP coordinator also supervises the lunchroom and chats with the students on the BEP at that time as well.

WHAT IF STAFF ARE NOT IMPLEMENTING THE BEP CORRECTLY?

All staff should receive inservice training on the purpose of the BEP, the positive nature of the program, and how to provide feedback to students. At times, teachers will write negative comments on the DPR. Some teachers may misuse it as a tool to punish students by writing down all of the inappropriate behaviors in which students engaged. Some teachers may need individual training and follow-up to reemphasize the positive nature of the program and to provide prompts for positive feedback. Many schools we have worked with have a line for teacher feedback on the DPR that prompts them to write positive rather than negative comments. For example, one school we worked with had a schoolwide positive reinforcement system in which students would receive "Wow!" tickets for following schoolwide expectations. In this school, the word "Wow!" was written next to the line for additional teacher feedback on the DPR. This provided teachers with a visual reminder to provide positive feedback and was consistent with schoolwide acknowledgment systems.

One way to keep the system positive and teachers invested in it is to make sure they are receiving feedback, at least quarterly, on how students on the BEP are doing. One thing that happens frequently in schools is that the teacher helps in the data collection process (e.g., filling out ODR forms for students engaging in severe or dangerous behavior or completing the DPR), but never sees a summary of the data or how the data are used to make decisions in schools. Staff should be updated on how many students are served on the BEP, how many are meeting their goals on a regular basis, and other outcome data associated with BEP improvements (e.g., student improvements in grades and test scores).

As mentioned in Chapter 6, to keep the system positive, a school may also want to reward staff on a frequent basis for their participation in the BEP. For example, staff are required to initial DPRs for students participating in the BEP and are asked to write positive comments when appropriate. Teacher's names could be randomly selected from the student DPRs at monthly staff meetings to earn small prizes. Alternatively, prizes could be given for the most creative or encouraging comments written on student DPRs. Students on the BEP could also nominate staff members whom they felt helped them be successful on the BEP. These individuals could be recognized at a faculty meeting, assembly, or in the school newsletter.

HOW DO WE KNOW IF TEACHERS ARE GIVING CONSTRUCTIVE FEEDBACK AT APPROPRIATE TIMES?

The only way to know if teachers are giving feedback *at appropriate times* is to observe teachers in their classrooms. In many schools we work in, principals observe instruction on a regular basis and are examining the teacher's ability to manage behavior during this observation. It is during this time that principals will provide feedback to teachers on how the BEP is being implemented. Since this type of observation is less likely to happen on a regular basis due to the time and costs associated, there are other ways to check the constructiveness of teacher feedback.

One important sign is that the teacher is circling each individual number on the DPR at each period, rather than circling all numbers at the end of the day. When we examine DPRs, it is easy to spot which teachers have waited until the end of the day to score the student. Alternatively, you can directly ask the student how often she is receiving feedback. In some of our schools, the BEP coordinator is a paraprofessional who works with students in multiple school settings. This person can do spot-check observations of how the intervention is being implemented. In fact, some schools have developed a system that involves a person observing the teacher during the first few days of BEP implementation to make sure feedback is occurring at regular intervals. This is difficult for a paraprofessional to do but often a counselor or school psychologist can serve this function.

WHAT IF PARENTS OR CAREGIVERS ARE NOT FOLLOWING THROUGH, OR USE THE BEP AS A PUNITIVE SYSTEM?

One of the strengths of the BEP is the increased connection between home and school. Parents and caregivers are given daily feedback on how their child is doing in school. In some cases, we have had difficulty getting parents to follow through with reviewing the DPR nightly and providing positive feedback to the student. In these cases, we may call or meet with the parents to emphasize the importance of their participation. Many of the schools that we work with have parents, school staff, and students sign a "BEP Contract" agreeing to the responsibilities of participating in the BEP. This provides parents with clear expectations for the program and can be referred to to remind parents of their responsibilities.

An interesting finding from our research is that the parent element of the BEP tends to be the weakest element when examining fidelity of BEP implementation. Results from Hawken and Horner (2003) indicate that four of the critical features of the BEP (i.e., students checking in, regular teacher feedback, students checking out, and daily DPR data used for decision making) were implemented with an average of 87% fidelity across students. Parental feedback (i.e., signature on the DPR) was provided during only 67% of the fidelity implementation checks. It should be noted, however, that many of the students were successful on the BEP and were meeting daily point goals despite lack of parental participation. This finding has been replicated across several studies (e.g., Hawken, 2006; Hawken et al., 2007). Parental feedback is encouraged, but not necessary for student success on the BEP. There are many students who could benefit from the BEP who come from chaotic home environments. These students should be given equal opportunity to benefit from the BEP even if their parents are unable to participate. (Note: Parents should always still give permission for the student to participate in the BEP.)

There are unfortunate circumstances we have come across in schools in which students participating in the BEP are punished for having "bad days." A bad day may mean that the student has not met his or her goal for that day. Some parents have implemented harsh punishments (e.g., spanking, hitting, yelling, extreme limitation of activities) when the DPR was brought home and the student had not done as well as expected. School staff typically hear about this from the student, or the student stops wanting to participate in the BEP. In these instances schools have set up "surrogate parents" at the school who serve as the additional person who provides feedback, praise, and comments on the DPR. The surrogate parent could be a teacher (other than the student's regular teacher), custodian, paraprofessional, or volunteer who is in the school daily, or some other adult who can commit 5 minutes each day to reviewing the student's DPR and providing positive feedback. The issue of harsh punishment will need to be addressed with the parent and would probably be best handled by having either the counselor, principal, or vice principal meet with the parent.

WHAT IF A STUDENT IS CONSISTENTLY PARTICIPATING IN THE BEP, AND HIS OR HER BEHAVIOR GETS WORSE?

It is expected that within about 2 weeks, students' behavior should improve on the BEP. For students who are receiving support to improve academic outcomes, it may take longer to notice changes in grades, but there should be an increase in organization, homework completion, and the like. Students whose behavior gets worse may need a more intensive, individualized intervention. Additional assessment data can be taken using functional behavioral assessment procedures. It is likely that classroom observations will be included when gathering information. Once information is gathered, it is used to develop an individualized behavior support plan. For more information on functional behavioral assessment and behavior support planning, refer to Crone and Horner (2003).

FINAL COMMENTS ON BEP IMPLEMENTATION

The BEP is an effective intervention, but it requires deep commitment from school staff and a focus on prevention. In our experience, there are several factors that indicate schools will have a difficult time implementing the BEP. These factors are listed below.

Schools will struggle with BEP implementation if:

- The administrator is not a member of the team that *develops* the BEP and *examines data* for decision making.
- The BEP is used as punishment rather than as a prevention program.

  - For example: "You have six ODRs and your punishment is the BEP."
  - The DPR is used as a means for teachers to vent their frustrations about challenging students.

- The BEP coordinator lacks skills to implement the program.

  - Skills are needed in behavior intervention, managing multiple students, and data entry/using computers.
  - See training needed for BEP coordinator in Chapter 5.

- Schools expect the BEP to solve all behavior problems.

  - Schools need several interventions at the Tier II level to support students at risk.
  - Schools need good academic supports and ability to identify escape behavior.
  - Schools need intensive interventions for students who are not successful with the BEP.

- Evaluation of BEP data is not embedded into existing teams, with a focus on alterable variables versus unalterable ones (e.g., poor parenting practices).

Appendices

CHAPTER 6

CHAPTER 7

CHAPTER 8

CHAPTER 9

List of Acronyms and Definitions

BEP. Behavior Education Program. The BEP is a daily check-in/check-out system that provides the student with immediate feedback on his or her behavior (via teacher rating on a Daily Progress Report) and increased positive adult attention.

BSP. Behavior Support Plan. An individualized plan to address a student's behavioral goals and objectives. The BSP should describe the intervention strategies to be used, the person responsible for implementation, a timeline for implementation, and the means by which the outcomes of the BSP will be evaluated.

DPR. Daily Progress Report. The DPR is the form used in the Behavior Education Program to track a student's daily progress toward meeting his or her behavioral goals. Samples of several DPRs are provided in the Appendices.

ELL. English language learner. An ELL student is a student whose native language is not English. ELL students are often provided with language support and instruction through placement in ELL classrooms or programs.

FBA. Functional behavioral assessment. An assessment of a person's behavior that is based on determining the function that the behavior serves for that person. The assessment typically consists of interviews with teachers, the student, and parents, as well as observations of the student's behavior in the problematic setting. The information gained from the FBA is used to develop a hypothesis regarding the purpose of the student's behavior and the circumstances under which the behavior occurs. The assessment information is used to build an individualized behavior support plan for that student.

IEP. Individualized education plan. An IEP describes the educational program that has been designed to meet the needs of any student who receives special education and related services. Each IEP should be a truly individualized document. The document identifies the student's needs, goals, and objectives, and strategies that will be implemented in the school to meet those objectives. Frequency and duration of the strategies should be included as well.

ODR. Office discipline referral. A system used in many schools to send a student to the main office to receive consequences following a behavioral infraction in the classroom or other social setting. The ODR refers to the documentation of that incident.

Working Smarter, Not Harder Organizer

Committee, project, or initiative	Purpose	Outcome	Target group	Staff involved

Request for Assistance Form

Date: _____   Teacher/Team: _____

Student name: _____   Grade: _____   IEP: Yes   No   (Circle)

1. Check the area(s) of concern:

Problem behavior	Academic problems	What is your primary concern?
___ Aggressive ___ Noncompliant ___ Disruptive ___ Withdrawn ___ Tardy ___ Lack of social skills ___ Other (specify) _____ _____	___ Reading ___ Math ___ Spelling ___ Writing ___ Study skills ___ Organization	

2. Check the strategies you have tried so far:

General review	Modify environment or teaching	Teach expected behaviors	Consequences tried
___ Review cumulative file ___ Talk with parents ___ Talk with previous teacher ___ Seek peer help ___ Classroom assessment ___ Other (specify) _____ _____	___ Change seating arrangement ___ Provide quiet space ___ Encourage work breaks ___ Change schedule of activities ___ Modify assignments ___ Arrange tutoring to improve student's academic skills ___ Other (specify) _____ _____	___ Give reminders about expected behavior when problem behavior is likely ___ Self-management program ___ Clarify rules and expected behavior for whole class ___ Practice expected behaviors in class ___ Contract with students ___ Other (specify) _____ _____	___ Increase rewards for expected behavior ___ Phone call to parents ___ Office referral ___ Time-out ___ Reprimand ___ Lunch detention ___ Loss of privileges ___ Meeting with parents ___ Other (specify) _____ _____

(cont.)

3. Why do you believe the student is engaging in problem behavior?

___ Adult attention   ___ Peer attention   ___ Escape from difficult work/tasks

___ Escape from peers   ___ Escape from adults

___ Gain access to preferred activity/item (computers, games, toys, etc.)

Teacher gathers:

- *Academic performance data*—DIBELS/CBM, percent of in-class/homework completion, documentation of grade-level performance
- *Behavior data*—behavior logs, documentation of in-class consequences, interclass time-outs

Front office gathers:

SWIS _____   Attendance _____   Tardies _____

    (# of ODRs)   (# of absences)   (# of tardies)

Parental Permission Form

Permission for Behavior Education Program (BEP)

Date: _____

Student: _____ Grade: _____

Teacher: _____

Parent/Guardian: _____

I would like to include your child in our BEP intervention. A report will be filled out daily by the teacher(s) and checked at the end of the day by our BEP coordinator, _____. Students will need to pick up their report every morning between _____ and _____ A.M. and then return to _____ between _____ and _____ P.M. The student will be able to earn incentives and rewards for appropriate behavior. As parents, you are responsible for making sure your child arrives on time each day for check-in and that you review and sign the daily progress report. Together, we can make this a positive experience for your child.

_____ I **do** give consent for my student to participate.

_____ I **do not** give consent for my student to participate.

_____ Date: _____
                        (Parent/Guardian)

For further information, please call:

_____ at: _____
                    (Coordinator)

or call: _____.

Daily Progress Report—Middle School, Example 1

A- Day   B-Day

Name: _____   Date: _____

Teachers: Please indicate Yes (2), So-So (1), or No (0) regarding the student's achievement for the following goals.

Goals	1/5			2/6			3/7			HR			4/8		
Be respectful	2	1	0	2	1	0	2	1	0	2	1	0	2	1	0
Be responsible	2	1	0	2	1	0	2	1	0	2	1	0	2	1	0
Keep hands and feet to self	2	1	0	2	1	0	2	1	0	2	1	0	2	1	0
Follow directions	2	1	0	2	1	0	2	1	0	2	1	0	2	1	0
Be there— be ready	2	1	0	2	1	0	2	1	0	2	1	0	2	1	0
TOTAL POINTS															
TEACHER INITIALS															

BEP Daily Goal   / 50   BEP Daily Score   / 50

In training _____   BEP Member _____   _____
                                                 Student signature

Teacher comments: Please state briefly any specific behaviors or achievements that demonstrate the student's progress. (If additional space is required, please attach a note and indicate so below.)

Period 1/5 _____

Period 2/6 _____

Period 3/7 _____

Homeroom _____

Period 4/8 _____

Parent/Caregiver Signature: _____

Parent/Caregiver Comments: _____

_____

Daily Progress Report—Middle School, Example 2

Name: _____

Materials to Class	Worked and Let Others Work	Follow Directions the First Time		Teacher	Parent
2 1 No	2 1 No	2 1 No	Assignments: Wow,		
2 1 No	2 1 No	2 1 No	Assignments: Wow,		
2 1 No	2 1 No	2 1 No	Assignments: Wow,		
2 1 No	2 1 No	2 1 No	Assignments: Wow,		
2 1 No	2 1 No	2 1 No	Assignments: Wow,		

Thumbs-Up! Ticket

THUMBS UP! TICKET

Student name: _____

Issued by: _____

Date: _____

WAY TO GO!

Daily Progress Report—Elementary School, Example 1

Name: _____

Date: _____

| 2 = **Wow!** |
| 1 = **OK** |
| 0 = **Tough time** |

GOALS		8:15–Recess	Recess–Lunch	Lunch–Recess	Recess–2:50
Be Safe	• Walk in building • Keep hands and feet to self	0 1 2	0 1 2	0 1 2	0 1 2
Be Respectful	• Follow directions	0 1 2	0 1 2	0 1 2	0 1 2
	• Use kind words and actions	0 1 2	0 1 2	0 1 2	0 1 2
Be Responsible	• Take care of myself and my belongings • Be in the right place and be ready	0 1 2	0 1 2	0 1 2	0 1 2
	Teacher Initials _____				

Total Points = _____ Points Possible = _____

Today _____ % Goal _____ %

Way to Be: _____

Parent Signature: _____

203

Daily Progress Report—Elementary School, Example 2

Date: _____

Teacher: _____   Student: _____

0 = No	1 = Good	2 = Excellent

	Be Safe	Be Respectful	Be Your Personal Best		
	Keep hands, feet, and objects to self	Use kind words and actions	Follow directions	Work in class	Teacher initials
9:00–A.M. Recess	0 1 2	0 1 2	0 1 2	0 1 2	
A.M. Recess–Lunch	0 1 2	0 1 2	0 1 2	0 1 2	
Lunch–P.M. Recess	0 1 2	0 1 2	0 1 2	0 1 2	
P.M. Recess–3:40	0 1 2	0 1 2	0 1 2	0 1 2	
Total Points = Points Possible = 50		Today _____%		Goal _____%	

Parent Signature: _____

WOW: _____

BEP Implementation Readiness Questionnaire

Is your school ready to implement the BEP? Prior to implementation of the BEP, it is recommended that the following features be in place. Please circle the answer that best describes your school at this time.

Yes   No   1. Our school has a schoolwide positive behavior support system in place. In essence, we have decided on three to five rules and have explicitly taught the rules to all students. We provide rewards to students for following the rules and mild consequences for rule infractions.

Yes   No   2. We have secured staff commitment for implementation of the BEP. The majority of staff agree that this intervention is needed to support students at risk for serious problem behavior, and they are willing to actively participate in the intervention.

Yes   No   3. There is administrative support for implementation of the BEP intervention. The administrative staff are committed to implementing and maintaining the BEP in our school. Administrators have allocated the necessary financial and staff resources to support implementation of the program.

Yes   No   4. There have been no major recent changes in the school system that could hinder successful implementation of the BEP intervention. Major changes include things such as teacher strikes, high teacher or administrative turnover, or major changes in funding.

Yes   No   5. We have made implementation of the BEP one of the school's top three priorities for this school year.

APPENDIX C.2

Voting Form for Implementing the BEP Intervention

☐ **YES**, I would be willing to participate in the Behavior Education Program intervention if it were implemented in our school as part of our schoolwide behavior support program.

☐ **NO**, I would *not* be willing to participate in the Behavior Education Program intervention if it were implemented in our school as part of our schoolwide behavior support program.

Questions, comments, or concerns: ______________________________

____

____

____

____

____

____

BEP Development and Implementation Guide

1. Determine personnel needs and logistics.
   - Who will be the BEP coordinator?

   - Who will supervise the BEP coordinator?

   - Who will check students in and out when coordinator is absent? (Name **at least two** people who can substitute for the coordinator.)

   - Where will check-in and check-out occur?

   - What is the maximum number of students that can be served on the BEP at one time?

   - What is the name of the BEP at your school and what will the Daily Progress Report be called?

2. Develop a Daily Progress Report (DPR).
   - What will the behavioral expectations be?

     - Consistent with schoolwide expectations?

   - Are the expectations positively stated?

   - Is the DPR teacher-friendly? How often are teachers asked to rate the student's behavior?

   - Is the DPR age-appropriate and does it include a range of scores?

   - Are the data easy to summarize?

(cont.)

3. Develop a reinforcement system for students on the BEP.
   - What will the students daily point goal be?

   - What reinforcers will students receive for checking in (e.g., praise and lottery ticket)?

   - What reinforcers will students receive for checking out **AND** meeting their daily point goal?

   - How will you ensure students do not become bored with the reinforcers?

   - What are the consequences for students who receive major and minor referrals?

4. Develop a referral system.
   - How will students be referred to the BEP? What are the criteria for placing students on the BEP?

   - What does the parental consent form look like for students participating in the BEP?

   - What is the process for screening students who transfer into the school?

   - What is the process for determining whether students will begin the next school year on the BEP?

5. Develop a system for managing the daily data.
   - Which computer program will be used to summarize data?

   - Which team in the school will examine the daily BEP data and how frequently will it be examined? (Note: data should be examined at least twice-monthly.)

   - Who is responsible for summarizing the data and bringing it to team meetings?

(cont.)

- How frequently will data be shared with the whole staff?

- How frequently will data be shared with parents?

6. Plan to fade students off the intervention.
   - What are the criteria for fading students off the BEP?

   - How will the BEP be faded and who will be in charge of helping students fade off the BEP?

   - How will graduation from the BEP be celebrated?

   - What incentives and supports will be put in place for students who graduate from the program?

7. Plan for staff training.
   - Who will train staff on the BEP?

   - Who will provide teachers with individual coaching if the BEP is not being implemented as planned?

   - Who will provide yearly booster sessions about the purpose and key features in implementing the BEP?

8. Plan for student and parent training.
   - Who will meet with students to train them on the intervention?

   - How will parents be trained on the intervention?

BEP Check-In, Check-Out Form—Elementary School

Student	Check-out (% of points earned)	Goal	Check-in	Delivered contract	Signed parent copy of DPR

BEP Check-In, Check-Out Form—Middle/High School

Date: _____   BEP coordinator: _____

| | Check-in | | | | Check-out |
Student name	Paper	Pencil	Notebook	BEP parent copy	% of points earned

Reinforcer Checklist

(To be completed by the student)

Please circle YES or NO if the item or activity is something you would like to earn.

Activity Reinforcers

Video game	YES	NO	Basketball	YES	NO
Swimming	YES	NO	Magazine	YES	NO
Watching video/DVD	YES	NO	Drawing	YES	NO
Walking	YES	NO	Field trips	YES	NO
Comic books	YES	NO	Puzzles	YES	NO
Play-Doh	YES	NO	Board game	YES	NO
Craft activities	YES	NO	Card game	YES	NO

Please list any other favorite activities you would like to earn.

_____

_____

_____

Material Reinforcers

Stickers	YES	NO	Erasers	YES	NO
Special pencils	YES	NO	Bubbles	YES	NO
Lotions	YES	NO	Play-Doh	YES	NO
Colored pencils/crayons	YES	NO	Rings	YES	NO
Free tardy pass	YES	NO	Puzzles	YES	NO
Bookmarks	YES	NO	Trading cards	YES	NO
Action figures	YES	NO	Small toys	YES	NO
Free assignment pass	YES	NO	Necklaces	YES	NO

Please list any other favorite items you would like to earn.

_____

_____

_____

(cont.)

Reinforcer Checklist *(page 2 of 2)*

Edible Reinforcers

Small one-bite candies	YES	NO	Cereal	YES	NO
Larger candy	YES	NO	Fruit	YES	NO
Vending machine drink	YES	NO	Pretzels	YES	NO
Juice/punch	YES	NO	Potato chips	YES	NO
Vegetables and dip	YES	NO	Corn chips	YES	NO
Crackers	YES	NO	Cookies	YES	NO
Donuts	YES	NO	Bagels	YES	NO
Candy bars	YES	NO	Cheese	YES	NO

Please list any other favorite name brands or snacks you would like to earn.

____

____

____

Social Reinforcers

Pat on the back	YES	NO	Verbal praise	YES	NO
Extra P.E./gym time	YES	NO	Free time	YES	NO
Games with teacher	YES	NO	Field trips	YES	NO
Games with friends	YES	NO	Special seat	YES	NO
Lunch with friends	YES	NO	High 5	YES	NO
Visit with friends	YES	NO	Awards	YES	NO

Please list any other favorites you would like to earn.

____

____

____

BEP Fidelity of Implementation Measure (BEP-FIM)

Scoring Guide

School: _____ Date: _____ Pre: _____ Post: _____

District: _____ State: _____ Data collector: _____

Evaluation Question	Data Source (P = permanent product; I = interview; O = observation)	Score (0–2)
1. Does the school employ a BEP coordinator whose job is to manage the BEP with 10–15 hours per week allocated? (0 = no BEP coordinator, 1 = BEP coordinator but less than 10 hours per week allocated, 2 = BEP coordinator, 10–15 hours per week allocated)	Interviews with administrator and BEP coordinator **I**	
2. Does the school budget contain an allocated amount of money to maintain the BEP (money for reinforcers, DPR forms, etc.)? (0 = no, 2 = yes)	BEP budget **P/I** Interviews	
3. Do students who are referred to the BEP receive support within a week of the referral? (0 = more than 2 weeks between referral and BEP support, 1 = within 2 weeks, 2 = within a week)	Interviews **P/I** BEP referrals and BEP start dates	
4. Does the administrator serve on the behavior support team or review BEP data on a regular basis? (0 = no, 1 = yes, but not consistently, 2 = yes)	Interviews **I**	
5. Do 90% of BEP team members state that the BEP system has been taught/reviewed on an annual basis? (0 = 0–50%, 1 = 51–89%, 2 = 90–100%)	Interviews **I**	
6. Do 90% of the students on the BEP check in daily (randomly sample 3 days for recording)? (0 = 0–50%, 1 = 51–89%, 2 = 90–100%)	BEP Check-In, **P** Check-Out Form	
7. Do 90% of students on the BEP check out daily (randomly sample 3 days for recording)? (0 = 0–50%, 1 = 51–89%, 2 = 90–100%)	BEP Check-In, **P** Check-Out Form	
8. Do 90% of students on the BEP report that they receive reinforcement (e.g., verbal, tangible) for meeting daily goals? (0 = 0–50%, 1 = 51–89%, 2 = 90–100%)	Interviews with **I** students on BEP	

(cont.)

Evaluation Question	Data Source (P = permanent product; I = interview; O = observation)		Score (0–2)
9. Do 90% of students on the BEP receive regular feedback from teachers (randomly sample 50% of student DPRs across 3 days)? (0 = 0–50%, 1 = 51–89%, 2 = 90–100%)	BEP Daily Progress Reports	P	
10. Do 90% of students on the BEP receive feedback from their parents? (0 = 0–50%, 1 = 51–89%, 2 = 90–100%)	BEP Daily Progress Reports	P	
11. Does the BEP coordinator enter DPR data at least once a week? (0 = no, 1 = every other week, 2 = once a week)	Interviews	I	
12. Do 90% of behavior support team members indicate that the daily BEP data is used for decision making? (0 = 0–50%, 1 = 51–89%, 2 = 90–100%)	Interviews	I	

BEP Acceptability Questionnaire—Teacher Version

_____ has been on the BEP since _____.

For each statement, **circle one number** that best describes how you feel about the BEP.

1. Problem behaviors have decreased since enrollment in the BEP.

Strongly disagree					Strongly agree
1	2	3	4	5	6

2. Appropriate classroom behaviors have increased since enrollment in the BEP.

Strongly disagree					Strongly agree
1	2	3	4	5	6

3. It was relatively easy (e.g., amount of time/effort) to implement the BEP.

Strongly disagree					Strongly agree
1	2	3	4	5	6

4. How effective was the BEP in decreasing this student's number of absences and tardies?
(This question does not apply. This student is rarely tardy or absent. Check here _____.)

Not effective					Very effective
1	2	3	4	5	6

5. The BEP process for this student was worth the time and effort.

Strongly disagree					Strongly agree
1	2	3	4	5	6

6. I would recommend that other schools use the BEP process with similar students.

Strongly disagree					Strongly agree
1	2	3	4	5	6

7. Please list any other comments or concerns.

BEP Acceptability Questionnaire—Student Version

For each statement, **circle one number** that best describes how you feel about the BEP.

1. The BEP helps improve my behavior **at school.**

   Strongly disagree   Strongly agree

   1   2   3   4   5   6

2. The BEP helps **increase** my homework completion and classroom assignments completion.

   Strongly disagree   Strongly agree

   1   2   3   4   5   6

3. The BEP helps **decrease** the number of days I am tardy.
   (This question does not apply to me. I am rarely tardy. Check here _____.)

   Strongly disagree   Strongly agree

   1   2   3   4   5   6

4. The BEP helps **decrease** the number of days I am absent.
   (This question does not apply to me. I am rarely absent. Check here _____.)

   Strongly disagree   Strongly agree

   1   2   3   4   5   6

5. It is easy to be on the BEP (carry the DPR around, get DPR signed by parent[s], check in and check out daily, etc.).

   Strongly disagree   Strongly agree

   1   2   3   4   5   6

6. The BEP is worth the time and effort. Overall, it really helps me.

   Strongly disagree   Strongly agree

   1   2   3   4   5   6

7. If I had a choice, I would participate in the BEP again.

   Strongly disagree   Strongly agree

   1   2   3   4   5   6

8. I think the BEP would be good for other kids who may be struggling in school.

   Strongly disagree   Strongly agree

   1   2   3   4   5   6

BEP Acceptability Questionnaire—Parent Version

For each question or statement, **circle one number** that best indicates how you feel about the BEP.

1. How effective was the BEP in improving your child's behavior **at school?**

   Not effective   Very effective

   1   2   3   4   5   6

2. How effective was the BEP in increasing your child's academic performance (e.g., improving his or her grades)?

   Not effective   Very effective

   1   2   3   4   5   6

3. How effective was the BEP in decreasing your child's number of absences and tardies?
   (This question does not apply. My child is rarely tardy or absent. Check here _____.)

   Not effective   Very effective

   1   2   3   4   5   6

4. How easy is it to participate in the BEP (e.g., review and sign DPR, attend meetings)?

   Very difficult   Very easy

   1   2   3   4   5   6

5. Having my child on the BEP is worth my time and effort.

   Strongly disagree   Strongly agree

   1   2   3   4   5   6

6. The BEP really helps me know how well my child is doing in school on a daily basis.

   Strongly disagree   Strongly agree

   1   2   3   4   5   6

7. I would recommend the BEP to other parents and students.

   Strongly disagree   Strongly agree

   1   2   3   4   5   6

BEP Contract

I, _____ , agree to work on these things this year.

1. _____

2. _____

3. _____

I will work with _____ to keep track of my progress.
I understand that I will have a chance to earn a reward each week when I meet my goals. A list of
rewards I would like to earn include:

1. _____

2. _____

3. _____

I will try hard to do my best to meet these goals every day.

_____
Signature of Student

I will do my best to help _____ meet his/her goals every day.

_____   _____
Signature of Coordinator   Signature of Parent

BEP Support Plan

Name: _____ Date of support request: _____ Grade: _____

Parent's name: _____ Parent's phone no: _____

Requested by: _____

Reason for request: _____

Functional Behavioral Assessment Activites

Step 1: Gather Information (Give dates of completion)

Parent Contact _____ Staffing _____ Observation (optional) _____

FBA Interview _____ Student Interview (optional) _____

IEP: ___ Yes ___ No No. of office referrals: _____ No. of absences: _____

Step 2: Propose a Summary Statement of the Problem

What sets off the problem?	What are the problems?	Why are they happening?

Step 3: Propose Appropriate BEP Options

☐ Basic BEP ☐ Modified BEP ☐ Individualized Support ☐ Other

(cont.)

Design Support Plan

Step 4: Conduct BEP Team Meetings to Determine Student Goal and Design Plan

Student Goal: _____

_____

Additional Supports	When	Where	Who Responsible

Step 5: Conduct Review Meetings and Use Student Monitoring Form to Monitor Progress

BEP Student Monitoring Form

Student Name: _____   Facilitator Name: _____

Student Goal: _____

Date	Additional Supports Completed	To do next • Continue • Modify • Monitor	Student's Progress

Functional Behavioral Assessment—Behavior Support Plan Protocol (F-BSP Protocol)

FUNCTIONAL BEHAVIORAL ASSESSMENT INTERVIEW—TEACHER/STAFF/PARENT

Student name: _____ Age: _____ Grade: _____ Date: _____

Person(s) interviewed: _____

Interviewer: _____

Student Profile: What is the student good at or what are some strengths that the student brings to school?

_____

_____

Step 1: Interview Teacher/Staff/Parent

Description of the Behavior

> **What does the problem behavior(s) look like?**
>
> **How often does the problem behavior(s) occur?**
>
> **How long does the problem behavior(s) last when it does occur?**
>
> **How disruptive or dangerous is the problem behavior(s)?**

Description of the Antecedents
Identifying Routines: When, where, and with whom are problem behaviors most likely?

Schedule (Times)	Activity	Specific Problem Behavior	Likelihood of Problem Behavior		With Whom Does Problem Occur?
			Low High 1 2 3 4 5 6		
			1 2 3 4 5 6		
			1 2 3 4 5 6		
			1 2 3 4 5 6		
			1 2 3 4 5 6		
			1 2 3 4 5 6		
			1 2 3 4 5 6		

(cont.)

Summarize Antecedents (and Setting Events)

What situations seem to set off the problem behavior? (difficult tasks, transitions, structured activities, small-group settings, teacher's request, particular individuals, etc.)

When is the problem behavior most likely to occur? (times of day and days of the week)

When is the problem behavior least likely to occur? (times of day and days of the week)

Setting Events: Are there specific conditions, events, or activities that make the problem behavior worse? (missed medication, history of academic failure, conflict at home, missed meals, lack of sleep, history of problems with peers, etc.)

Description of the Consequences

What ususally happens after the behavior occurs? (what is the teacher's reaction, how do other students react, is the student sent to the office, does the student get out of doing work, does the student get in a power struggle, etc.)

- - - - - - End of Interview - - - - - -

Step 2: Propose a Testable Explanation

Setting Events	Antecedents	Behaviors	Consequences
		1.	
		2.	

Function of the Behavior

For each ABC sequence listed above, why do you think the behavior is occurring? (to get teacher attention, peer attention, desired object/activity, or escape undesirable activity, demand particular people, etc.)

1. _____

2. _____

How confident are you that your testable explanation is accurate?

Very sure			So-so		Not at all sure
6	5	4	3	2	1

(cont.)

INSTRUCTIONS FOR COMPLETING THE FUNCTIONAL BEHAVIORAL ASSESSMENT— BEHAVIOR SUPPORT PLAN PROTOCOL (F-BSP PROTOCOL)

The F-BSP Protocol was designed as a tool to guide the process of completing a functional behavioral assessment (FBA) and of linking the assessment to the design of an individual behavior support plan (BSP). The F-BSP Protocol is divided into eight Steps: (1) Interview Teacher/Staff/Parent/Student; (2) Propose a Testable Explanation; (3) Rate Your Confidence in the Testable Explanation; (4) Conduct Observations; (5) Confirm/Modify Testable Explanation; (6) Build a Competing Behavior Pathway; (7) Select Intervention Strategies; and (8) Evaluation Plan.

The F-BSP Protocol can be used to complete either a simple FBA or a full FBA. In a simple FBA, Steps 4 and 5 are omitted. The Student Interview portion of Step 1 is omitted as well in a simple FBA.

Demographic Information

Before any interview, it is important to explain the purpose of the interview to the interviewee. Spend a little time explaining why you are doing the interview, indicate that you think it will take about 20–30 minutes to complete, and note that you will follow up with the interviewee once the FBA is completed.

Take a few minutes to complete the demographic information at the top of page 1. For confidentiality purposes, you may choose to use only the student's initials or to identify the student by his or her student number.

In the space next to "Person(s) interviewed," indicate the person's relationship to the student (math teacher, lunchroom monitor, parent, etc). In the space next to "Interviewer," indicate the interviewer's role in the behavior support process (action team member, team leader, school psychologist, etc.).

In the space next to "Student Profile," ask the interviewee to list some of the student's strengths, skills, or talents. Also list items or activities that the student enjoys or will work for. This information will help you to design a BSP that builds on the student's strengths and that includes consequences that are personally reinforcing to the student.

Step 1: Interview Teacher/Staff/Parent

The purpose of Step 1 is to get a clear understanding of the problem behavior(s) of concern and to identify routines that predict or support the problem behavior. This is accomplished by generating a clear definition of the problem behavior, and by identifying the setting events, antecedents, and consequences of the problem behavior.

The first interview should be conducted with the person who made the initial request for assistance. This may be the student's primary teacher or any other adult with whom the student has significant contact (e.g., the lunchroom monitor, school counselor, or algebra teacher). A simple FBA typically includes only one teacher interview. A full FBA may include additional interviews with relevant adults, including other teachers or a parent. Copies of the teacher/staff/parent interview can be made to accommodate the need for multiple interviews.

(cont.)

Description of the Behavior

The interviewer asks the interviewee four questions regarding the problem behavior.

1. What does the problem behavior(s) look like?
2. How often does the problem behavior(s) occur?
3. How long does the problem behavior(s) last when it does occur?
4. How disruptive or dangerous is the problem behavior?

Write down the answers to each question in the space provided. Prompt the interviewee to be as specific as possible. If the answer to the question is not specific, measurable, or observable, prompt the interviewee to be clearer in his or her response. For example, in response to question 1, the interviewee may say, *"Marisa is spacey and distractible in class."* This definition of the problem behavior is unclear— "spacey and distractible" may mean something different to the interviewer than it does to the interviewee. Prompt the interviewee by saying, *"How do you know when Marisa is being spacey and distractible? What does it look like?"* Continue to prompt the interviewee until the description of the problem behavior is clear enough that two observers would be able to recognize it independently. If the interviewee describes more than one problem behavior in question 1, be sure to get answers to questions 2, 3, and 4 for each problem behavior. Make a clear note of this on the interview form.

Description of the Antecedents

An *antecedent* is an event or circumstance that happens before a behavior occurs. It can be thought of as the predictor of a problem behavior. Examples of antecedents that could set off problem behavior include asking the student to do a demanding or long task; placing the student next to another child whom he or she dislikes; or expecting a student to complete a task during unstructured work time. The same antecedent could set off problem behavior for one student, while it helps another student to perform successfully. Because antecedents can vary so much among different students, it is very important to understand the antecedents that matter to the student with whom you are concerned. You can begin to identify the antecedents to problem behavior by looking at the student's daily routine.

Begin by completing the table on the bottom of page 1. In the first two columns, fill in the student's daily schedule. In the first column, indicate the time period for the activity, and in the second column briefly describe the activity. For example, for a middle school student you would write down the time for first period and the name of the class that the student has during first period. Then you would continue on through the last period of the day. The schedule for an elementary school student can be obtained from the student's primary teacher. An elementary school schedule is usually broken into smaller time periods, by subject or activity (e.g., math, science, circle time). The interview will go quicker if you can get the child's schedule and complete this section before you begin the interview. If you are interviewing a parent, you will complete the first two columns of this table a little differently. Ask the parent to think of the times of his or her day that are related to school. Some examples include getting ready for school in the morning, transportation to school, transportation home from school, and doing homework. Include all of these activities in the "Activity" column. Ask the parent to provide you with a general idea of times when these activities occur.

Complete the rest of the table for the time periods you have listed. Look at the first time period. Ask the interviewee if the student engages in problem behavior during that time period. If he or she does, ask the interviewee what type of problem behavior occurs. Write this down in the column marked "Specific Problem Behavior." The problem behaviors that you write down should reflect the problem behaviors that you discussed in the first section of the interview. You should already have a good description of these behaviors, so it is fine to write a brief description in this column (e.g., you could write "temper tantrum," "fighting," or "distractible" because these behaviors are specifically described in the first section).

(cont.)

After you have written down the type of problem behavior that occurs during a time period, ask the interviewee how likely it is that the problem behavior will occur during that time period. Ask him or her to rate the likelihood on a scale of 1 to 6, where 1 means that it rarely happens and 6 means that it happens on a daily basis. Circle that number in the next column.

Finally, ask the interviewee with whom the problem is most likely to occur. Does the student get into trouble with other students? Is the student defiant toward the teacher? Perhaps the problem does not impact anyone other than the student. In this column, indicate if the problem occurs with peers, teacher, self, parent, or another significant person. If the interviewee indicates that the problem typically occurs with specific peers, you should indicate these students by using their initials only. Complete each of these columns for each time period listed.

Summarize Antecedents (and Setting Events)

The next section helps you to summarize and clarify the information you have learned from the description of the student's schedule. In this section, the interviewee will answer four questions:

1. What situations seem to set off the problem behavior?
2. When is the problem behavior most likely to occur?
3. When is the problem behavior least likely to occur?
4. Are there specific conditions, events, or activities that make the problem behavior worse?

To answer the first question, take a look at the completed table with the interviewee. First, look at the times when the student is most likely to engage in problem behavior—times when the likelihood is rated a 4, 5, or 6. Is there anything similar about those times? For example, is each time period an unstructured time, or do each of the time periods require the student to do demanding work on his or her own? Perhaps each is a time when the student's sibling is in the same class. Try to determine what is similar about the problematic routines that tend to set off the problem behavior. If the interviewee has trouble answering this question, prompt him or her by saying, *"If you wanted to make the problem behavior occur, what would you do?"*

Ask the interviewee what times of the day and days of the week the problem behavior is most likely to occur. If his or her answer is different than what you would expect (based on the information given in the schedule table), ask the interviewee to clarify his or her answer.

Ask the interviewee when the problem behavior is least likely to occur. Knowing when the problem behavior does not occur can help you identify things that work for the student. That is, there are some routines when the student does not get into trouble. If you can identify what it is about those routines that helps the student be successful, you can better determine how to change the student's unsuccessful routines.

Setting events are situations or circumstances that make it more likely that a problem behavior will occur or that make the problem behavior more intense. Some examples include: if the student has a fight with a parent right before coming to school, if the student didn't get enough sleep or missed a meal, or if the student misses taking medication. Ask the interviewee if he or she knows of certain situations that tend to make the student's problem behavior worse, or more likely to occur.

Description of the Consequences

In this section, you want to find out what usually happens after the problem behavior occurs. Is the student ignored or do all of his or her peers start to laugh? Is the student sent to the office? Is the student sent to time-out? Ask the interviewee what typically happens after the problem behavior occurs and what impact those consequences seem to have on the problem behavior. In other words, do the consequences make the problem behavior stop, improve, or get worse?

(cont.)

End of Interview

At this point, the face-to-face portion of the interview is completed. Next, you will summarize the information you have learned from the interview to create a "testable explanation" of why the problem behavior is occurring.

If you need to interview additional teachers or other adults (including parents), make copies of the first two pages of the F-BSP protocol and use the copies for as many interviews as you plan to conduct.

Step 2: Propose a Testable Explanation

ABC Sequence

A testable explanation is one of the most important pieces of the F-BSP process. It is the summary of everything you have learned about the problem behavior and the link to designing an effective, relevant BSP.

Begin to build your testable hypothesis by listing the problem behavior. It is likely that a student will engage in more than one type of problem behavior. For example, the same student might fight with other students and refuse to follow teacher directions. List each *type* of problem behavior separately in the column labeled "Behavior." (Don't list every single problem behavior displayed. For example, if fighting consists of pushing, hitting, and yelling at other students, you would lump all three behaviors into one *type* of behavior: "fighting.")

Next, for each type of behavior you have listed, indicate the antecedents that tend to set off or predict that behavior. List them under the column headed "Antecedents." Refer back to the interview information to identify the antecedents.

For each type of behavior you have listed, indicate the consequences that tend to support the problem behavior in the "Consequences" column. The interviewee will have told you about many potential consequences that occur. List the ones that seem to make the behavior continue or worsen. For example, a student who makes inappropriate jokes in class might encounter two consequences. First, the joke might be ignored by other students, and he is unlikely to tell that joke again. Second, he might get a lot of attention and laughter over his inappropriate joke. In that case, he is likely to tell other inappropriate jokes or tell the same joke in other classes. In this example, the ignoring consequence did not support the problem behavior, but the attention/laughter consequence did. For your testable explanation of why the problem behavior is occurring, you want to list the consequences that support the problem behavior. In the example, you would write "peer attention and laughter" under the column that is headed "Consequences."

Finally, if there are any setting events that make the problem behavior worse or more likely to occur, list them under the column headed "Setting Events."

Complete the Setting Events, Antecedents, and Consequences boxes for each *type* of behavior that you have listed. Each set of these is called an *ABC sequence.*

Function of the Behavior

For each ABC sequence, you want to determine why you think the behavior is occurring. At this point you can describe the behavior, you know what situations set it off, and you know what consequences make it continue or get worse. But why is the behavior happening? What function does it serve for the student? Some common functions include: to get peer attention, to get adult attention, to get out of doing difficult work, or to get away from someone the student doesn't like. For each ABC sequence, decide what you think is really motivating the problem behavior and write it down in the space provided.

Once you become more familiar with the F-BSP Protocol, it will become fairly easy to complete Step 2. At that point, we suggest that you complete Step 2 with the interviewee to check for his or her agreement with your summary of the interview.

Functional Assessment Checklist for Teachers and Staff (FACTS)

FACTS—Part A

<u>Step 1</u>

Student/Grade: _____ Date: _____

Interviewer: _____ Respondent(s): _____

<u>Step 2</u> **Student Profile: Please identify at least three strengths or contributions the student brings to school.**

_____

_____

<u>Step 3</u> **Problem Behavior(s): Identify problem behaviors**

___ Tardy	___ Inappropriate language	___ Disruptive	___ Theft
___ Unresponsive	___ Fight/physical aggression	___ Insubordination	___ Vandalism
___ Withdrawn	___ Verbal harassment	___ Work not done	___ Other _____

Describe problem behavior: _____

<u>Step 4</u> **Identifying Routines: Where, when, and with whom are problem behaviors are most likely?**

Schedule (Times)	Activity	With Whom Does Problem Occur?	Likelihood of Problem Behavior	Specific Problem Behavior
			Low High 1 2 3 4 5 6	
			1 2 3 4 5 6	
			1 2 3 4 5 6	
			1 2 3 4 5 6	
			1 2 3 4 5 6	
			1 2 3 4 5 6	
			1 2 3 4 5 6	

<u>Step 5</u> **Select one to three routines for further assessment. Select routines based on (1) similarity of activities (conditions) with ratings of 4, 5, or 6 and (2) similarity of problem behavior(s). Complete the FACTS—Part B for each routine identified.**

(cont.)

FACTS—Part B

Step 1 Student/Grade: _____ Date: _____

Interviewer: _____ Respondent(s): _____

Step 2 **Routine/Activities/Context: Which routine (only one) from the FACTS—Part A is assessed?**

Routine/Activities/Context	Problem Behavior

Step 3 **Provide more detail about the problem behavior(s):**

What does the problem behavior(s) look like?
How often does the problem behavior(s) occur?
How long does the problem behavior(s) last when it does occur?
What is the intensity/level of danger of the problem behavior(s)?

Step 4 **What are the events that predict when the problem behavior(s) will occur?**

Related Issues (Setting Events)		Environmental Features	
___ illness	Other: _____	___ reprimand/correction	___ structured activity
___ drug use	_____	___ physical demands	___ unstructured time
___ negative social	_____	___ socially isolated	___ tasks too boring
___ conflict at home	_____	___ with peers	___ activity too long
___ academic failure	_____	___ other	___ tasks too difficult

Step 5 **What consequences are most likely to maintain the problem behavior(s)?**

Things That Are Obtained		Things Avoided or Escaped From	
___ adult attention	Other: _____	___ hard tasks	Other: _____
___ peer attention	_____	___ reprimands	_____
___ preferred activity	_____	___ peer negatives	_____
___ money/things	_____	___ physical effort	

Step 6 **What current efforts have been used to control the problem behavior?**

Strategies for Preventing Problem Behavior		Consequences for Problem Behavior	
___ schedule change	Other: _____	___ reprimand	Other: _____
___ seating change	_____	___ office referral	_____
___ curriculum change	_____	___ detention	_____

SUMMARY OF BEHAVIOR

Step 7 **Identify the summary that will be used to build a plan of behavior support.**

Setting Events and Predictors	Problem Behavior(s)	Maintaining Consequence(s)

How confident are you that the Summary of Behavior is accurate?

Not very confident					Very confident
1	2	3	4	5	6

(cont.)

Instructions

The FACTS is a two-page interview used by school personnel who are building behavior support plans. The FACTS is intended to be an efficient strategy for initial functional behavioral assessment. The FACTS is completed by people (teachers, family, clinicians) who know the student best, and is used to either build behavior support plans, or to guide more complete functional assessment efforts. The FACTS can be completed in a short period of time (5–15 minutes). Efficiency and effectiveness in completing the forms increases with practice.

How to Complete the FACTS—Part A

Step 1: Complete Demographic Information

Indicate the name and grade of the student, the date the assessment data were collected, the name of the person completing the form (the interviewer), and the name(s) of the people providing information (respondents).

Step 2: Complete Student Profile

Begin each assessment with a review of the positive and contributing characteristics the student brings to school. Identify at least three strengths or contributions the student offers.

Step 3: Identify Problem Behaviors

Identify the specific student behaviors that are barriers to effective education, disrupt the education of others, interfere with social development, or compromise safety at school. Provide a brief description of exactly how the student engages in these behaviors. What makes his or her way of doing these behaviors unique? Identify the most problematic behaviors, but also identify any problem behaviors that occur regularly.

Step 4: Identify Where, When, and with Whom the Problem Behaviors Are Most Likely

A: List the times that define the student's daily schedule. Include times between classes, lunch, and before school, and adapt for complex schedule features (e.g., odd/even days) if appropriate.

B: For each time listed indicate the activity typically engaged in during that time (e.g., small-group instruction, math, independent art, transition).

C: Where appropriate indicate the people (adults and peers) with whom the student is interacting during each activity, and especially list the people the student interacts with when he or she engages in problem behavior.

D: Use the 1 to 6 scale to indicate (in general) which times/activities are most and least likely to be associated with problem behaviors. A "1" indicates low likelihood of problems, and a "6" indicates high likelihood of problem behaviors.

E: Indicate which problem behavior is *most likely* in any time/activity that is given a rating of 4, 5, or 6.

Step 5: Select Routines for Further Assessment

Examine each time/activity listed as 4, 5, or 6 in the table from Step 4. If activities are similar (e.g., activities that are unstructured; activities that involve high academic demands; activities with teacher reprimands; activities with peer taunting) and have similar problem behaviors, treat them as "routines for further analysis."

Select between one and three routines for further analysis. Write the name of the routine and the most common problem behavior(s). Within each routine identify the problem behavior(s) that are most likely or most problematic.

For *each* routine identified in Step 5 complete a FACTS—Part B.

(cont.)

How to Complete the FACTS—Part B

Step 1: Complete Demographic Information

Identify the name and grade of the student, the date that the FACTS—Part B was completed, who completed the form, and who provided information for completing the form.

Step 2: Identify the Target Routine

List the targeted routine and problem behavior from the bottom of the FACTS—Part A. The FACTS—Part B provides information about *one* routine. Use multiple Part B forms if multiple routines are identified.

Step 3: Provide Specifics about the Problem Behavior(s)

Provide more detail about the features of the problem behavior(s). Focus specifically on the unique and distinguishing features, and the way the behavior(s) is disruptive or dangerous.

Step 4: Identify Events That Predict Occurrence of the Problem Behavior(s)

Within each routine what (1) setting events and (2) immediate preceding events predict when the problem behavior(s) will occur? What would you do to make the problem behavior(s) happen in this routine?

Step 5: Identify the Consequences That May Maintain the Problem Behavior

What consequences appear to reward the problem behavior? Consider that the student may get/obtain something he or she wants, or that he or she may escape/avoid something he or she finds unpleasant.

Identify the *most powerful* maintaining consequence with a "1," and other possible consequences with a "2" or "3." Do not check more than three options. The focus here is on the consequence that has the greatest impact.

When problems involve minor events that escalate into very difficult events, separate the consequences that maintain the minor problem behavior from the events that may maintain problem behavior later in the escalation.

Step 6: Define What Has Been Done to Date to Prevent/Control the Problem Behavior

In most cases, school personnel will have tried some strategies already. List events that have been tried, and organize these by (1) those things that have been done to prevent the problem from getting started, and (2) those things that were delivered as consequences to control or punish the problem behavior (or reward alternative behavior).

Step 7: Build a Summary Statement

The summary statement indicates the setting events, immediate predictors, problem behaviors, and maintaining consequences. The summary statement is the foundation for building an effective behavior support plan. Build the summary statement from the information in the FACTS—Part A and FACTS—Part B (especially the information in Steps 3, 4, and 5 of the FACTS—Part B). If you are confident that the summary statement is accurate enough to design a plan, move into plan development. If you are less confident, then continue the functional assessment by conducting direct observation.

High School BEP Referral Form

Student: _____ Date: _____

Grade: _____ Counselor: _____

Referral submitted by: _____ Class: _____

1. Student strengths: _____

2. Is the student qualified for special education services?   Y   N

3. How many days has the student been suspended this year? _____

4. Please give an estimate of student's academic progress in your classroom:

    _____ (classwork)

    _____ (homework)

    _____ (test average)

Problem behavior(s): Identify Top Three Most Problematic Behaviors

___Tardy	___Fight/physical aggression	___Disruptive	___Theft
___Unresponsive	___Inappropriate language	___Insubordination	___Vandalism
___Withdrawn	___Verbal harassment	___Incomplete work	___Other _____
	___Verbally inappropriate	___Self-injury	_____

What have you tried? _____

_____

_____

How has it worked? _____

_____

_____

Why do you think the behavior(s) keep happening? _____

_____

_____

_____

High School Daily Plan Agenda

Activity	Directions
Planner check	Get out your planner! Open to today's date.
Daily entry task	Using your planner, make a list of all the homework you have due within the next 3 days. Pick the most difficult homework assignment. Make a list of what you need to complete this homework (time, assistance, worksheet, etc.). (5 minutes)
Homework completion session	After you complete the daily entry task start the homework you identified as the most difficult. Discuss what you need with teacher as he/she comes around the room for the planner check. (40 minutes)

Reinforcer Checklist for High School BEP

(To be completed by the student)

Please circle YES or NO to if the item or activity is something you would like to earn.

Activity Reinforcers

Working online	YES	NO	Magazine	YES	NO
Working with a peer	YES	NO	Drawing	YES	NO
Watching video/DVD	YES	NO	Board game	YES	NO
Choice of class activity	YES	NO	Puzzles	YES	NO
Listening to music	YES	NO	Reading	YES	NO

Please list any additional favorite activities that you would like to earn.

_____

_____

_____

_____

Material Reinforcers

Art supplies	YES	NO	Parking pass	YES	NO
Colored pencils/crayons	YES	NO	Thumbdrive	YES	NO
Lotion/lip gloss	YES	NO	Backpack	YES	NO
School lanyard	YES	NO	Sports tickets	YES	NO
Sudoku/crossword puzzles	YES	NO	Dance tickets	YES	NO
Free assignment pass	YES	NO	Coffee card	YES	NO

Please list any additional favorite items that you would like to earn.

_____

_____

_____

_____

(cont.)

Reinfocer Checklist for High School BEP *(page 2 of 2)*

Edible Reinforcers

Juice box	YES	NO	Cereal	YES	NO
Gum	YES	NO	Fruit	YES	NO
Pretzels	YES	NO	Cheese	YES	NO
Potato chips	YES	NO	Granola bar	YES	NO
Vegetables and dip	YES	NO	Corn chips	YES	NO
Crackers	YES	NO	Cookies	YES	NO
Mini-pizza	YES	NO	Bagels	YES	NO

Please list any additional favorite name brands or special foods that you may enjoy.

____

____

____

____

Social Reinforcers

Class assistant	YES	NO	Verbal praise	YES	NO
Extra P.E./gym time	YES	NO	Awards	YES	NO
Lunch with teacher	YES	NO	Field trips	YES	NO
Lunch with friends	YES	NO	Special seat	YES	NO
Update to favorite teacher	YES	NO	Call parents	YES	NO
Extra art time	YES	NO	Class reward	YES	NO
"Star" in PBS video	YES	NO			

Please list any additional favorite activities that you would like to earn.

____

____

____

____

References

Alberto, P. A., & Trautman, A. C. (2006). *Applied behavior analysis for teachers* (7th ed.). Columbus, OH: Merrill.

Blum, C. (2006). *Staff development and the validity of measures for schoolwide positive behavior supports.* Paper presented at the International Positive Behavior Support Conference, Reno, NV.

Bohanon-Edmonson, H., Flannery, K. B., Eber, L., & Sugai, G. (Eds.). (2005). *Positive behavior support in high schools: Monograph from the 2004 Illinois High School Forum of Positive Behavior Interventions and Supports* (rev.). Retrieved July 22, 2007, from *www.pbis.org/files/PBSMonographComplete.pdf.*

Campbell, S. B. (1998). Development perspectives. In T. H. Ollendick & M. Hersen (Eds.), *Handbook of child psychopathology* (3rd ed., pp. 3–35). New York: Plenum Press.

Chafouleas, S. M., Christ, T. J., Riley-Tillman, T. C., Briesch, A. M., & Chanese, J. M. (2007). Generalizability and dependability of daily behavior report cards to measure social behavior of preschoolers. *School Psychology Review, 36*(1), 63–79.

Chafouleas, S. M., Riley-Tillman, T. C., Sassu, K. A., LaFrance, M. J., & Patwa, S. S. (2007). Daily behavior report cards (DBRCs): An investigation of consistency of on-task data across raters and method. *Journal of Positive Behavior Interventions, 9,* 30–37.

Cheney, D., Blum, C., & Walker, B. (2004). An analysis of leadership teams' perceptions of positive behavior support and the outcomes of typically developing and at-risk students in their schools. *Assessment for Effective Intervention, 30,* 7–24.

Chinien, C., & Boutin, F. (2001). Qualitative assessment of cognitive-based dropout prevention strategy. *High School Journal, 85,* 1–11.

Christenson, S. L., Sinclair, M. F., Lehr, M. F., & Hurley, C. M. (2000). Promoting successful school completion. In K. M. Minke & G. C. Bear (Eds.), *Preventing school problems, promoting school success: Strategies and programs that work* (pp. 211–257). Bethesda, MD: National Association of School Psychologists.

Colvin, G., Kameenui, E. J., & Sugai, G. (1993). School-wide and classroom management: Reconceptualizing the integration and management of students with behavior problems in general education. *Education and Treatment of Children, 16,* 361–381.

Conroy, M. A., Davis, C. A., Fox, J. J., & Brown, W. H. (2002). Functional assessment of behavior and effective supports for young children with challenging behavior. *Assessment for Effective Instruction, 27,* 35–47.

Crone, D. A., & Horner, R. H. (2003). *Building positive behavior support systems in schools: Functional behavioral assessment.* New York: Guilford Press.

Crone, D. A., Horner, R. H., & Hawken, L. S. (2004). *Responding to problem behavior in schools: The Behavior Education Program.* New York: Guilford Press.

Croninger, R. G., & Lee, V. E. (2001). Social capital and dropping out of high school: Benefits to at-risk students of teachers' support and guidance. *Teachers College Record, 103*(4), 548–581.

Davies, D. E., & McLaughlin, T. F. (1989). Effects of a daily report on disruptive behaviour in primary students. *BC Journal of Special Education, 13,* 173–181.

Dodge, D. T., & Colker, L. (2002). *The creative curriculum* (5th ed.). Washington, DC: Teaching Strategies.

Dougherty, E. H., & Dougherty, A. (1977). The daily report card: A simplified and flexible package for classroom behavior management. *Psychology in the Schools, 14*(2), 191–195.

Elliot, S. N., & Gresham, F. M. (1991). *Social skills intervention guide: Practical strategies for social skills training.* Circle Pines, MN: American Guidance Service.

Fairbanks, S., Sugai, G., Guardino, D., & Lathrop, M. (2007). Response to intervention: Examining classroom behavior support in second grade. *Exceptional Children, 73*(3), 288–310.

Fairchild, T. N. (1987). The daily report card. *Teaching Exceptional Children, 19*(2), 72–73.

Filter, K. J., McKenna, M. K., Benedict, E. A., Horner, R. H., Todd, A. W., & Watson, J. (2007). Check in/check out: A post-hoc evaluation of an efficient, secondary-level targeted intervention for reducing problem behaviors in schools. *Education and Treatment of Children, 30*(1), 69–84.

Flannery, K. B., McGrath Kato, M., Fenning, P., & Bohanon, H. (in press). Office discipline referral patterns in high schools implementing School-wide Positive Behavior Support (SWPBS): Preliminary findings. *Journal of School Violence.*

Forgan, J. W., & Vaughn, S. (2000). Adolescents with and without LD make the transition to middle school. *Journal of Learning Disabilities, 33,* 33–43.

Fox, L., Dunlap, G., & Cushing, L. (2002). Early intervention, positive behavior support, and transition to school. *Journal of Emotional and Behavioral Disorders, 10*(3), 149–157.

Good, R. H., & Kaminski, R. A. (Eds.). (2001). *Dynamic Indicators of Basic Early Literacy Skills* (6th ed.). Eugene, OR: Institute for the Development of Educational Achievement.

Gresham, F. M., & Elliot, S. N. (1990). *Social skills rating system.* Circle Pines, MN: American Guidance Service.

Hawken, L. S. (2006). School psychologists as leaders in the implementation of a targeted intervention: The Behavior Education Program (BEP). *School Psychology Quarterly, 21,* 91–111.

Hawken, L. S., & Adolphson, S. L., MacLeod, K. S., & Schumann, J. (2009). Secondary tier interventions and supports. In G. Sugai, R. H. Horner, G. Dunlap, & W. Sailor (Eds.), *Handbook of positive behavior support* (pp. 391–416). New York: Springer.

Hawken, L. S., & Horner, R. H. (2003). Evaluation of a targeted intervention within a school-wide system of behavior support. *Journal of Behavioral Education, 12,* 225–240.

Hawken, L. S., MacLeod, K. S., & Rawlings, L. (2007). Effects of the Behavior Education Program (BEP) on problem behavior with elementary school students. *Journal of Positive Behavior Interventions, 9,* 94–101.

Hawken, L. S., & O'Neill, R. E. (2006). Including students with severe disabilities at all levels of school-wide positive behavioral support. *Research and Practice for Persons with Severe Disabilities, 31,* 46–53.

Hawken, L. S., Pettersson, H., Mootz, J., & Anderson, C. (2005). *The Behavior Education Program: A check-in, check-out intervention for students at risk [DVD].* New York: Guilford Press.

Hertzog, C. J., & Morgan, P. L. (1999). Making the transition from middle level to high school. *High School Magazine, 6*(4), 26–30.

Horner, R. H., Sugai, G., Todd, A. W., & Lewis-Palmer, T. (2005). School-wide positive behavior support. In L. Bambara & L. Kern (Eds.), *Individualized supports for students with problem behaviors: Designing positive behavior plans* (pp. 359–390). New York: Guilford Press.

Horner, R. H., Todd, A. W., Lewis-Palmer, T., Irvin, L. K., Sugai, G., & Boland, J. B. (2004). The School-Wide Evaluation Tool (SET): A research instrument for assessing school-wide positive behavior support. *Journal of Positive Behavior Interventions, 6,* 3–12.

Kea, C. D., & Utley, C. A. (1998). To teach me is to know me. *Journal of Special Education, 32*(1), 44–47.

Kincaid, D. (2007, March). *Response to Intervention and PBS.* Paper presented at the International Positive Behavior Support Conference, Boston, MA.

Klump, J., & McNeir, G. (2005). *Culturally responsive practices for student success: A regional sampler.* Portland, OR: Northwest Regional Educational Laboratory. Retrieved November 20, 2007, from *www.nwrel.org/request.*

Lane, K. L., Wehby, J., Menzies, H. M., Doukas, G. L., Munton, S. M., & Gregg, R. M. (2003). Social skills instruction for students at risk for antisocial behavior: The effects of small-group instruction. *Behavioral Disorders, 28*(3), 229–248.

Lawry, J., Danko, C., & Strain, P. (1999). Examining the role of the classroom environment in the prevention of problem behaviors. In S. Sandall & M. Ostrosky (Eds.), *Young exceptional children monograph series: Practical ideas for addressing challenging behaviors* (pp. 49–61). Longmont, CO: Sorpis West.

Leach, D. J., & Byrne, M. K. (1986). Some "spill-over" effects of a home-based reinforcement programme in secondary school. *Educational Psychology, 6*(3), 265–276.

Lenz, B. K., & Deshler, D. D. (1998). *Teaching content to all: Evidence-based inclusive practices in middle and secondary schools.* Boston: Allyn & Bacon.

Lewis, T. J., & Sugai, G. (1999). Effective behavior support: A systems approach to proactive school-wide management. *Effective School Practices, 17*(4), 47–53.

March, R. E., & Horner, R. H. (2002). Feasibility and contributions of functional behavioral assessment in schools. *Journal of Emotional and Behavioral Disorders, 10*(3), 158–170.

May, S., Ard, W. III, Todd, A. W., Horner, R. H., Glasgow, A., Sugai, G., et al. (2000). *Schoolwide information system.* Eugene, OR: Educational and Community Supports, University of Oregon. Available at *www.swis.org.*

McCurdy, B. L., Kunsch, C., & Reibstein, S. (2007). Secondary prevention in the urban school: Implementing the Behavior Education Program. *Preventing School Failure, 51*(3), 12–19.

McIntosh, K., Flannery, K. B., Sugai, G., Braun, D., & Cochrane, K. L. (2008). Relationships between academics and problem behavior in the transition from middle school to high school. *Journal of Positive Behavior Interventions, 10*, 243–255.

Mizelle, N. B., & Irvin, J. L. (2000). Transition from middle school into high school. *Middle School Journal, 31*(5), 37–61.

Morrison, G. M., Anthony, S., Storino, M., & Dillon, C. (2001). An examination of the disciplinary histories and the individual and educational characteristics of students who participate in an inschool suspension program. *Education and Treatment of Children, 24*, 276–293.

Nelson, J. R. (1997). *Designing schools to enhance the academic and social outcomes of all students* (Report No. R305F6011). Washington, DC: Department of Education. (ERIC Document Reproduction Service No. ED410516)

Newman, B. M., Lohman, B. J., Newman, P. R., Myers, M. C., & Smith, V. L. (2000). Experiences of urban youth navigating the transition to ninth grade. *Youth and Society, 31*, 387–416.

O'Neill, R. E., Horner, R. H., Albin, R. W., Sprague, J. R., Storey, K., & Newton, J. S. (1997). *Functional assessment for problem behavior: A practical handbook* (2nd ed.). Pacific Grove, CA: Brooks/Cole.

OSEP Technical Assistance Center on Positive Behavioral Interventions and Supports. (n.d.). *Schoolwide PBS: Secondary prevention.* Retrieved February 18, 2005, from *www.pbis.org/secondaryprevention.htm.PB.*

Osher, D., Dwyer, K., & Jackson, S. (2004). *Safe, supportive and successful schools step by step.* Longmont, CO: Sopris West.

Powers, L. J. (2003). *Examining the effects of targeted group social skills intervention in schools with and without school-wide systems of positive behavior support.* Unpublished doctoral dissertation, University of Missouri, Columbia.

Roeser, R. W., & Eccles, J. S. (2000). Schooling and mental health. In A. J. Sameroff, M. Lewis, & S. M. Miller (Eds.), *Handbook of developmental psychopathology* (2nd ed., pp. 135–156). New York: Kluwer Academic/Plenum.

Shinn, M. R. (1989). *Curriculum-based measurement: Assessing special children.* New York: Guilford Press.

Sinclair, M. F., Christenson, S. L., Evelo, D. L., & Hurley, C. M. (1998). Dropout prevention for youth with disabilities: Efficacy of a sustained school engagement procedure. *Exceptional Children, 65*(1), 7–21.

Sinclair, M. F., Christenson, S. L., Lehr, C. A., & Anderson, A. R. (2003). Facilitating student engagement: Lessons learned from Check & Connect longitudinal studies. *California School Psychologist, 8,* 29–41.

Sue, D. W., Carter, R. T., Casas, J. M., Fouad, N. A., Ivey, A. E., & Jensen, M. (1998). *Multicultural counseling competencies: Individual and organizational development* (Vol. 11). Thousand Oaks, CA: Sage.

Sugai, G., & Horner, R. H. (1999). Discipline and behavioral support: Preferred processes and practices. *Effective School Practices, 17*(4), 10–22.

Sugai, G., & Horner, R. H. (2002a). The evolution of discipline practices: School-wide positive behavior supports. *Child and Family Behavior Therapy, 24,* 23–50.

Sugai, G., & Horner, R. H. (2002b). Introduction to the special series on positive behavior support in schools. *Journal of Emotional and Behavioral Disorders, 10,* 130–135.

Swanson, H. L., & Deshler, D. D. (2003). Instructing adolescents with learning disabilities: Converting a meta-analysis to practice. *Journal of Learning Disabilities, 36*(2), 124–135.

Taylor-Greene, S., Brown, D., Nelson, L., Longton, J., Gassman, T., Cohen, J., et al. (1997). School-wide behavioral support: Starting the year off right. *Journal of Behavioral Education, 7,* 99–112.

Todd, A. W., Kaufman, A., Meyer, G., & Horner, R. H. (2008). The effects of a targeted intervention to reduce problem behaviors: Elementary school implementation of check in–check out. *Journal of Positive Behavioral Interventions, 10,* 46–55.

Tyack, D. (2001). Introduction. In S. Mondale & S. Patton (Eds.), *School: The story of American public education* (pp. 1–10). Boston: Beacon Press.

Walker, H. M., & Horner, R. H. (1996). Integrated approaches to preventing antisocial behavior patterns among school age children and youth. *Journal of Emotional and Behavioral Disorders, 4*(4), 194–210.

Walker, H. M., Horner, R. H., Sugai, G., Bullis, M., Sprague, J. R., Bricker, D., et al. (1996). Integrated approaches to preventing antisocial behavior patterns among school-age children and youth. *Journal of Emotional and Behavioral Disorders, 4,* 194–209.

Walker, H. M., Kavanagh, K., Stiller, B., Golly, A., Severson, H. H., & Feil, E.G. (1998). First Step to Success: An early intervention approach for preventing school failure. *Journal of Emotional Behavior Disorders, 4*(2), 66–80.

Walker, H. M., Ramsey, E., & Gresham, F. M. (2004). *Antisocial behavior in school: Evidence-based practices* (2nd ed). Belmont, CA: Thomson Wadsworth.

Walker, H. M., & Severson, H. (1992). *Systematic screening of behavior disorders (SSBD): A multiple gating procedure.* Longmont, CO: Sopris West.

Warberg, A., George, N., Brown, D., Chauran, K., & Taylor-Greene, S. (1995). *Behavior Education Plan handbook.* Elmira, OR: Fern Ridge Middle School.

Index

Page numbers followed by an *f* or *t* indicate figures or tables.

240